Assessing Race, Ethnicity and Gender in Health

Assessing Race, Ethnicity and Gender in Health

Sana Loue

Case Western Reserve University
Cleveland, Ohio

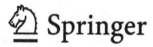 Springer

Sana Loue
Case Western Reserve University
Cleveland, OH 44106–4945
USA

Cover illustration © *2010 Superstock*

ISBN 978-1-4419-4080-3
e-ISBN 0-387-32462-3
e-ISBN 978-0-387-32462-3

Printed on acid-free paper.

Printed in the United States of America.   (TB/MVY)

9 8 7 6 5 4 3 2 1

springer.com

Acknowledgments

This book would not have been possible without the vision of my former editor, Mariclaire Cloutier, and my current editor, Bill Tucker. Appreciation is due to a number of individuals for their assistance with the research. Gary Edmunds, Nancy Mendez, Ingrid Vargas, and Jenice Contreras deserve recognition for the many hours that they spent tracking down references.

I owe special thanks to members of the communities with which I work, too numerous to name individually, for their contributions to my education and to the evolution of my understanding of identities.

List of Tables

1. Comparison of categories and definitions for race and ethnicity developed by Federal Office of Management and Budget 27

2. Comparison of three approaches to color classification in Nicaragua 28

3. Diagnostic criteria and symptoms for gender identity disorders 68

4. Classification systems of bisexuality 74

5. Selected studies indicating prevalence of sexual behavior in comparison with sexual identity 76

6. Estimated AIDS cases by race/ethnicity 91

7. Summary table of selected measures of ethnic and racial identity and identification 121

8. Summary table of selected measures of immigration status 124

9. Characteristics of selected measures of acculturation 128

10. Summary table of selected tools to assess gender role 138

11. Summary table of suggested dimensions of assessment for sexual orientation 146

Contents

Prologue   xi

PART I   FOUNDATIONS

1. Constructing Categories: Context and Consequences   3
2. Methodological Considerations...   11

PART II   CONSTRUCTS: THEIR DEFINITION AND USE

3. Defining Race, Ethnicity and Related Constructs.......................   25
4. Defining Sex, Gender, and Sexual Orientation Constructs.............   54
5. Race, Ethnicity, and Sexual Orientation in Health.....................   86

PART III   ASSESSING GENDER, ETHNICITY, AND RELATED
           CONSTRUCTS

6. Measures of Ethnicity, Ethnic Identification, Acculturation,
   and Immigration Status..   119
7. Measures of Sex, Gender, Gender Role, and Sexual Orientation......   136

Index   153

Prologue

American studies are five times more likely than European trials to report in publications the race or ethnicity of the study participants (Sheikh, Netuveli, Kai, and Panesar, 2004). In a review of full-length articles appearing in three major pediatric journals, for instance, it was found that over one-half of the published reports contained data on participants' race and/or ethnicity (Walsh and Ross, 2003). Nearly 80% of hospitals in the United States collect data on race and ethnicity (Runy, 2004). Despite the relatively high prevalence of collecting and reporting race/ethnicity information, however, significant debate continues regarding the wisdom of this practice. The following objections have been voiced with regard to the collection and use of data relating to race and ethnicity.

- The categories once used are inadequate and categories change too frequently to make the collection of the data worthwhile. As an example, during the period from 1990 to 2003, hospitals in Rhode Island utilized three different classification systems for the collection and recording of race and ethnicity data (Buechner, 2004).
- Categories that we construct may not be valid due to intermarriage. The most recent census data indicates that over 2% of the American population, or more than 7 million persons, now acknowledge a multiracial identity (Ahmann, 2005). Children were more likely to be recorded as having a multiracial identity than adults, which suggests an increase in interracial coupling.
- Data collection based on self-reports is not valid because individuals change their self-identification depending upon the context in which they are asked to so designate (Kaplan and Bennett, 2003).
- Individuals grouped into the same category demonstrate significant genetic diversity, so that the construction of the categories is questionable (Erickson, 2003; Schultz, 2003). There are no gene variants that are present in all individuals of one population and that are absent in the individuals of another population group (Bonham, Warshauer-Baker, and Collins, 2005). For instance, Wilson and colleagues (2001) found in a study of drug-metabolizing enzymes and genotyping in eight populations around the world that genotypes clustered into four groups,

but the four groups did not correspond to the populations from which they had been drawn.

- Categorizations are too broad to have any definitive medical meaning (Schultz, 2003) and may obscure heterogeneity within groups (Kaufman, 1999; Williams, 2001). Gatrad and Sheikh (2000) have cautioned health care providers to refrain from making assumptions about patients' willingness or unwillingness to undergo particular screening tests or elective procedures on the basis of their ethnicity.
- Socially determined categories cannot be applied to biological science (Schultz, 2003).
- Classifying individuals on the basis of socially constructed categories of race and ethnicity serves to reinforce racial and ethnic divisions that already exist (Azuonye, 1996; Bogue and Edwards, 1971; Fullilove, 1998; Stolley, 1999).
- The categories developed for race and ethnicity are often used to compare minority groups to the majority population and these comparisons often focus on the negative aspects of the health and lives of minority group members (López, 2003).
- A focus on ethnic or racial groups may lead researchers to believe or encourage them to disregard relevant social or cultural processes that are shared across group boundaries (Garro, 2001).

Additional concerns have been voiced with regard to the assessment of acculturation level and immigration status, two constructs that are relevant to race and ethnicity.

- Categories of immigration status change too frequently to be useful over time. As an example, attempts to assess immigrants' utilization of publicly funded health care for specific services must be cognizant of the fluctuations in participants' eligibility for benefits as a result of changes in their immigration status and/or changes in the relevant legislation (Loue, Cooper, and Lloyd, 2005).
- Self-reports of immigration status will be inaccurate, if they are provided, due to fears of deportation.
- Questions relating to immigration status will result in poor recruitment and retention due to fears of the consequences that might ensue following disclosure.

Similar objections have been raised to the collection of data relating to sexual orientation and sexual identity:

- Sexual orientation and/or sexual identity are fluid over a lifetime and assessment at one point in time may be inaccurate.
- How an individual chooses to identify him- or herself may not be reflective of his or her true orientation because of concern about the consequences of self-disclosure and, accordingly, collection of this information is not valuable.
- Assessment of sexual orientation tends to compare homosexuals and heterosexuals, with the resulting inference that homosexuality is somehow "less than" or "worse than" or undesirable.

Indeed, with respect to any or all of these variables, there is little consensus among researchers as to how categories should be defined or who should be assigned to them. And, in view of such vociferous displeasure with the collection and recording of these variables in the context of health care and research, one must necessarily question why it is done.

Hospitals have been found to collect these data in order to meet the requirements of a law or regulation, to improve the quality of care, to ensure the availability of interpreter services, to improve or maintain community relations, to assist in targeting marketing efforts, and/or because it is perceived as beneficial (Runy, 2004). Pediatric researchers have reported collecting and reporting race and ethnicity data because it was required by the institutional review board of their institution, the National Institutes of Health, and/or the peer-reviewed journal in which they wished to publish; to conform to a tradition of reporting race and ethnicity data; to better describe the study population; and/or because they believed that it was relevant (Walsh and Ross, 2003).

Scholars have suggested other reasons underlying the necessity for the collection of data relating to race and ethnicity (Mays, Ponce, Washington, and Cochran, 2003). These reasons are relevant, as well, to data regarding sexual orientation.

(1) To describe vital and health statistics. These data provide information that can be utilized by public health programming and planning to develop programs targeting specific health issues of concern in a manner that is appropriate to the affected communities.

(2) To identify risk indicators for specific health outcomes. It has been argued that ethnicity itself constitutes a risk factor for specific diseases, such as Tay-Sachs, which occurs predominantly in individuals of Eastern European Jewish descent (Greenidge, 2004). Alleles associated with sickle cell anemia are not evenly distributed across racial/ethnic groups, but are found more frequently in African-American populations (Collins, 2004). The risk factor profile for breast cancer among African-American women has been found to differ from that of white women, although the underlying mechanisms of these differences require further investigation (Bernstein, Teal, Joslyn, and Wilson, 2003).

(3) To improve the delivery of health care services (Hasnaian-Wynia and Pierce, 2005). Nonwhite patients have been found to rate the quality of and their satisfaction with their health care lower than do whites (Haviland, Morales, Reise, and Hays, 2003). To some extent, this difference may be attributable to disparate treatment by health care providers associated with differences in patient self-identified or perceived race or ethnicity (Bach, Pham, Schrag, Tate, and Hargraves, 2004; van Ryn and Burke, 2000).

(4) To identify markers of unmeasured biological differences. Researchers have reported slower metabolism of some drugs in persons of Asian ethnicity, compared to white and blacks (Meadows, 2003). It has been hypothesized that this difference may be attributable, in part, to genetic factors that have not yet been identified.

(5) To identify proxy variables for unmeasured social factors. Race, ethnicity, sex, and sexual orientation may serve as markers for other variables that we are unable

to identify due to limitations in our knowledge and/or the methodologies available to us.

Accordingly, if we are to collect these data, we must confront and address numerous challenges. These include issues of operationalization of these constructs in a manner that is appropriate to the research question and the study and target populations, measurement, and sampling. Ethical issues are also raised by our construction of these categories that must be addressed if we are to remain respectful of the communities with which we work.

This text addresses many of these issues. Part I focuses on the foundations underlying the development of these categories and brings to the fore important ethical and methodological issues in their construction and their use. Part II provides a review of the literature that offers definitions of these constructs and their use in health research. Examples of research that has relied on categories of race, ethnicity, and/or sexual orientation are provided, with commentary that discusses the appropriateness of their use and the conclusions that were drawn as a result. The final portion of the text provides a summary of many measures currently available to assess race, ethnicity, sexual orientation, and related constructs.

References

Ahmann, E. (2005).Tiger Woods is not the only "Cablinasian": Multi-ethnicity and health care. *Pediatric Nursing* 31(2): 125–129.

Azuonye, I.O. (1996). Guidelines will encourage the thinking that underpins racism in medicine. *British Medical Journal* 313: 426.

Bach, P.B., Pham, H.H., Scrag, D., Tate, R.C., Hargraves, J.L. (2004). Primary care physicians who treat blacks and whites. *New England Journal of Medicine* 351: 575–584.

Bernstein, L., Teal, C.R., Joslyn, S., Wilson, J. (2003). Ethnicity-related variation in breast cancer risk factors. *Cancer* 97 (1 Suppl): 222–229.

Bogue, G., Edwards, G.F. (1971). How to get along without race in demographic analysis. *Social Biology* 18: 387–396.

Bonham, V.L., Warshauer-Baker, E., Collins, F.S. (2005). Race and ethnicity in the genome era: The complexity of the constructs. *American Psychologist* 60(1): 9–15.

Buechner, J.S. (2004). Hospitalizations by race and ethnicity, Rhode Island, 1990–2003. *Medicine and Health/Rhode Island* 87(7): 220–221.

Collins, F.S. (2004). What we do and don't know about 'race', 'ethnicity', genetics and health at the dawn of the genome era. *Nature Genetics Supplement* 36(11): S13–S15.

Erickson, A.K. (2003). Ethnicity puts clinical trials to the test. *Nature Medicine* 9(8): 983.

Fullilove, M.T. (1998). Comment abandoning "race" as a variable in public health research: An idea whose time has come. *American Journal of Public Health* 88: 1297–1298.

Garro, L.C. (2001). The remembered past in a culturally meaningful life: Remembering as cultural, social, and cognitive processes. In C. Moore, H. Mathews (Eds.), *The Psychology of Cultural Experience* (pp. 105–147). U.K.: Cambridge University Press.

Gatrad, A.R., Sheikh, A. (2000). Birth customs: Meaning and significance. In A. Sheikh, A.R. Gatrad (Eds.), *Caring for Muslim Patients*. Oxford, UK: Radcliffe Medical Press Ltd.

Greenidge, K.C. (2005). Race, politics, ethnicity, and science. *American Journal of Ophthalmology* 139: 704–706.

Hasnaian-Wynia, R., Pierce, D. (2005). *HRET Disparities Toolkit: A Toolkit for Collecting Race, Ethnicity, and Primary Language Information from Patients*. The Health Research and Educational Trust. Available at http://www.hretdisparities.org. Last accessed November, 2005.

Haviland, M.G., Morales, L.S., Reise, S.P., Hays, R.D. (2003). Do health care ratings differ by race or ethnicity? *Joint Commission Journal on Quality and Safety* 29(3): 134–145.

Kaplan, J.B., Bennett, T. (2003). Use of race and ethnicity in biomedical publication. *Journal of the American Medical Association* 289(20): 2709–2716.

López, S.R. (2003). Reflections on the Surgeon General's Report on Mental Health, Culture, Race, and Ethnicity. *Culture, Medicine, and Psychiatry* 27: 419–434.

Loue S., Cooper, M., Lloyd L.S. (2005). Welfare and immigration reform and use of prenatal care among women of Mexican ethnicity in San Diego, California. *Journal of Immigrant Health* 7(1): 37–44.

Mays, V.M., Ponce, N.A., Washington, D.L., Cochran, S.D. (2003). Classification of race and ethnicity: Implications for public health. *Annual Review of Public Health* 24: 83–110.

Meadows, M. (2003). FDA issues guidance on race and ethnicity data. *FDA Consumer* May–June: 36.

Runy, L.A. (2004). Collecting race & ethnicity data. *Hospitals & Health Networks* 78(8): 30.

Sheikh, A., Netuveli, G., Kai, J., Panesar, S.S. (2004). Comparison of reporting of ethnicity in US and European randomised controlled trials. *British Medical Journal* 329 (7457): 87–88.

Schultz, J. (2003). FDA guidelines on race and ethnicity: Obstacle or remedy? *Journal of the National Cancer Institute* 95(6): 425–426.

Stolley, P.D. (1999). Race in epidemiology. *International Journal of Health Services* 29: 905–909.

Van Ryn, M., Burke, J. (2000). The effect of patient race and socio-economic status on physicians' perceptions of patients. *Social Science and Medicine* 50: 813–828.

Wash, C., Ross, L.F. (2003). Whether and why pediatric researchers report race and ethnicity. *Archives of Pediatric and Adolescent Medicine* 157: 671–675.

Wilson, J.F., Weale, M.E., Smith, A.C., Gratrix, F., Fletcher, B., Thomas, M.G., Bradman, N., Goldstein, D.B. (2001). Population genetic structure of variable drug response. *Nature and Genetics* 29(3): 265–269.

Part I
Foundations

1
Constructing Categories: Context and Consequences

The Social and Political Context of Categories

Increasingly, researchers, clinicians, policy makers, and others concerned with health and public health have focused their attention on disparities in access to health care, the quality of health care, and risk for various diseases across minority populations, which are often defined in terms of their race or ethnicity. These categories, however,

are human mental constructs . . . they are intellectual boundaries we put on the world in order to help us apprehend it and live in an orderly way . . . [N]ature doesn't have categories; people do (Stone, 1988: 307).

Categories have been distinguished from groups and classes. Jenkins (2003) has argued that the formation of groups and classes is rooted in the processes of internal definition, by which individuals signal to others both inside and outside of their group their self-definition of identity. These internal definitions and designations may be critical, depending upon the goals of a particular study. As an example, it may be important that a researcher studying social networks in the LGBT (lesbian, gay, bisexual, and transgender) communities understand how individuals self-classify because such distinctions establish their own position within a group and signal their group membership to others; these distinctions may, for instance, denote the degree of masculinity or femininity claimed, such as in the distinction made between butch and femme lesbians or bear and twinkie gay men. (For a discussion of some of these intra-group classifications, see Gibson and Meem, 2002; Stoller, 1991; Wright, 1997).

In contrast, categories are externally defined, although in actuality, the processes of defining the "us" and the "them" is an interactive one: the categorization of "them" assists in the definition of "us", while the definition of "us" is a function of the history of relationships with others (Hagendoorn, 1993; Jenkins, 2003). We form these categories based on perceived commonalities that we believe somehow distinguish those objects or persons that belong to a specified category and those that do not (Jay, 1981).

3

The process of categorizing may be effectuated in a number of ways (Jenkins, 2003). First, the external categorization of a group may coincide with one or more elements of the group's self-identification. Second, the categorization may be conducted by a group that the original group believes has the power and authority to so categorize them as a function of their superior knowledge, power, status, etc. This process of categorization is evident in the identification by scientists and researchers of those groups believed to be at increased risk of HIV infection during the early years of the epidemic in the United States. (See chapter 2). Third, the imposition of the categories may have been effectuated through the use of power that is exercised through the use of physical force or threat. The effective delineation in the United States between those who are black and those who are white on the basis of the "one drop rule" was implemented through the brutal institution of slavery in a legal context that permitted it. (See chapter 2). Finally, some groups may resist external categorization but the process of doing so requires the internalization of that categorization as the focus of denial. As an example, the rejection by homosexuals of their characterization by the American Psychiatric Association as different, and therefore mentally ill, by virtue of their sexual orientation requires the internalization of that differentness (although not the characterization as ill). Jenkins (2003: 69) has cautioned:

The effective categorization of a group of people by a more powerful 'other' is not therefore 'just' a matter of classification (if, indeed, there is such a thing). It is necessarily an inter-vention in that group's social world which will, to an extent and in ways that are a function of the specifics of the situation, alter that world and the experience of living in it.... [A] concern with external definition and categorization demands that we pay attention to *power* and *authority*, and the manner in which different modes of domination are implicated in the social construction of ethnic and other identities.... Unless we can construct an under-standing of ethnicity that can address *all* of ethnicity's facets and manifestations, from the celebratory communality of belonging to the final awful moment of genocide, we will have failed both ourselves and the people among whom we undertake our research.

Although scientists and researchers may not conceive of themselves as indi-viduals having power and authority, it is clear that as professionals they have significantly greater education, knowledge, status, and voice in relation to many of the groups who are the focus of research and, depending on context, the larger community as well. As such, they hold significant power and are often viewed as speaking with the voice of authority. This can be seen, for instance, in the re-lationship of the investigators to the research subjects in the Tuskegee syphilis experiment (see chapter 3), the previous characterization of homosexuality as a mental illness by the American Psychiatric Association (see discussion below), and the current classification of transsexuality as a mental disorder by that same association (see chapter 3). Freire (1970: 87) has addressed the significance of the labels that we assign:

Within the word we find two dimensions, reflection and action, in such radical interaction that if one is sacrificed—even in part—the other immediately suffers. There is no true word that is not at the same time a praxis. Thus, to speak a true word is to transform the world.

An unauthentic word, one which is unable to transform reality, results when dichotomy is imposed upon its constitutive elements.... Either dichotomy, by creating unauthentic forms of existence, creates also unauthentic forms of thought, which reinforce the original dichotomy.

We see, then, that how we construct our categories and labels frames our world, and that frame further reinforces our use of those categories. And, although our construction of categories varies and shifts over time, place, and purpose, we often act as if the categories to which we assign certain attributes and the members to whom we attribute these attributes are static and remain so. As an example, research indicates that the designation of an individual's race or ethnicity may vary over the course of his or her life depending upon who is charged with the responsibility or authority to make this designation: the individual's parent at the time of his or her birth, the individual him- or herself, the employer reporting on the composition of the workforce, and the coroner at the time of death (Yanow, 2003). Additionally, whether an individual self-identifies as a member of a particular group, whatever its nature, may vary depending upon the social, historical, and political context in which the designation is to be made.

Categories and Consequences: Ethical Implications

Not infrequently, this process of developing categories involves reference to a specific group that then becomes the category to which all others are compared. The construction of this referent category and the subsequent comparison of all other groups against this referent category may raise significant ethical issues. As one scholar stated, "If men define situations as real, they are real in their consequences" (Stone, 2003: 32, quoting W.I. Thomas).

The referent category often takes on a special significance in that it is isolated from all else [and] is A and pure. Not-A is necessarily impure, a random catchall, to which nothing is external except A and the principle of order that separates it from Not-A (Jay, 1981: 45).

As a result, members of those categories that are not-A, that are not part of the referent group and are perceived as different, also may be perceived as being deviant. This is best understood through an examination of the "social audience" approach to deviance.

The social audience approach defines who and what are deviant as a function of the viewers:

[W]hether or not an act is deviant depends on how others who are socially significant in power and influence define the act. One could commit any act, but it is not deviant in its social consequences if no elements of society react to it (Bell, 1971: 11).

[A]cts and actors violating the norms of society will be termed "rule-breaking behavior" and "rule breakers," while the terms "deviant behavior and "deviant" will be reserved for acts and actors labeled as deviant by a social audience (Cullen and Cullen, 1978: 8).

Kitsuse's view of deviance is particularly helpful in understanding how the categorization of individuals may lead to a perception of deviance:

Forms of behavior per se do not differentiate deviants from nondeviants; it is the responses of the conventional and conforming members of the society who identify and interpret behavior as deviant which sociologically transforms persons into deviants (Kitsuse, 1962: 253).

[D]eviance is not a property inherent in certain forms of behavior; it is a property conferred upon these forms by the audience which directly or indirectly witness them (Erikson, 1962: 308).

Ben-Yehuda (1990: 36) has asserted that "who interprets whose behavior, why, where, and when is very crucial . . . ." He offers two examples in support of his view. The first is that of Joan of Arc, who was executed in 1431 after having been convicted as a heretical deviant; she was later canonized by Pope Benedict XV. The second example is that of the Nobel Laureate chemist Louis Pauling. Pauling lobbied the United Nations during the late 1950s to end nuclear weapons testing. Despite the widespread support that he received from other scientists, his stance led to his interrogation by the U.S. Senate and a prohibition against his attendance at various international scientific meetings. In 1962, he was awarded the Nobel Peace Prize in recognition of his efforts to promote peace (Ben-Yehuda, 1990).

Depending upon the construction of the categories to be used in research and the portrayal of members of those groups, the construction of categories may also result in the marginalization of their members. Tucker (1990: 7) has defined marginalization as

the complex and disputatious process by means of which certain people and ideas are privileged over others at any given time . . . [and] the process by which, through shifts in position, any given group can be ignored, trivialized, rendered invisible and unheard, perceived as inconsequential, de-authorized, "other," or threatening, while others are valorized.

Marginalization and consequent devaluation may result when populations, groups, communities, or individuals do not conform to this idealized referent group. Marginalization may result from differences in gender (Amaro and Raj, 2000; Bauer, Rodriguez, Quiroga, and Flores-Ortiz, 2000), race and ethnicity (Gutierez and Lewis, 1997), social class (Marshall and McKeon, 1996), disability (Braithwaite, 1996), and/or sexuality (Corey, 1996; Yep and Pietri, 1999).

Consider, for example, intersexuality (discussed in greater depth in chapter 4). Epstein (1990: 104–105, 116) has argued that the medicalization of intersexuality altered

the social condition of hermaphrodites [when] the availability of surgical and pharmacological interventions could control or create a public sexual identity for these individuals. In mandating binary sex differentiation for legal purposes, medical jurisprudence has, then, imposed a clearcut distinction even though in biomedical terms such a distinction has been known not to exist . . . [T]he results of total medicalization return us to the semiotics of teratology: individuals with gender disorders are permitted to live, but the disorders themselves are rendered invisible, are seen as social stigmata to be excised in the operating room."

In this way, the adherence to a belief that humans must necessarily be biolog-ically of one sex or another reinforces and is then further reinforced by our con-struction of maleness and femaleness. We construct categories and then engage in activities to eliminate what is perceived to fall outside of these categories. We point to these categories that we have constructed as if they had naturally arisen and then proceed to interpret reality in the context of these "naturally-arising" categories.

A further example of the consequences of categorization of a group by those holding power and authority is provided by the previous psychiatric designation of homosexuality *per se* as a mental disorder. The second edition of the *Diagnostic and Statistical Manual* (1968), previously utilized by the American Psychiatric Association as a guide to the diagnosis of mental disorders, referred to homosexu-ality as a mental illness. The inclusion of homosexuality in this nosology removed it from the litany of behaviors that had previously fallen within the jurisdiction of the church as the guardian of morality and, to some extent, the legal system, which had viewed homosexuality as criminal in nature and therefore deserving of punishment (Bayer, 1981).

Accordingly, the psychiatric profession viewed itself as the protector "of de-viants who had suffered at the hands of society and the more traditional forces of social control" (Bayer, 1981:11). However, its increasing assumption of responsi-bility for the control of behaviors previously viewed as immoral and/or criminal, such as substance abuse and sexual deviance, was viewed by others as an attempt to widen the scope of its authority and foster a therapeutic state (Kittrie, 1972). Further, in the context of the civil rights movement of the 1960s and 1970s, ho-mosexuals began to see themselves as an oppressed minority that had been and continued to be oppressed by social institutions and ideological standards and began to campaign actively and vociferously to have homosexuality deleted as a class of mental illness (Bayer, 1981: 12–13). Bayer has explained the significance of this action:

To dismiss the significance of the debate over whether homosexuality ought to be included in the APA's nosological classification . . . is to miss the enormous importance it carried for American society, psychiatry, and the homosexual community. By investing the dispute with great meaning, the participants had themselves transformed it from a verbal duel into a crucial, albeit symbolic, conflict. The gay community understood quite well the social consequences of being labeled and defined by others, no matter how benign the posture of those making the classification. A central feature of its struggle for legitimation therefore entailed a challenge to psychiatry's authority and power to classify homosexuality as a disorder.

Gay organizations in New York City explained to the American Psychiatric Association in a memorandum:

We are told, from the time that we first recognize our homosexual feelings, that our love for other human beings is sick, childish and subject to "cure." We are told that we are emotional cripples forever condemned to an emotional status below that of the "whole" people who run the world. The result of this in many cases is to contribute to a self-image that often lowers the sights we set for ourselves in life, and many of us asked ourselves, "How could anybody love me?" or "How can I love somebody who must be just as sick as I am?" (Quoted in Bayer, 1981: 119).

Members of the psychiatric profession, too, campaigned for the elimination of homosexuality from the APA nosological classification. Thomas Szasz argued against the characterization of variance from behavioral norms as illnesses. Indeed, Szasz viewed the association of homosexuality with disease as a form of coercive social control (Bayer, 1981), recognizing the destructive consequences that resulted:

Psychiatric preoccupation with the disease concept of homosexuality—as with the disease concept of all so-called mental illnesses ... conceals the fact that homosexuals are a group of medically stigmatized and socially persecuted individuals. The noise generated by their persecution and their anguished cries of protest are drowned out by the rhetoric of therapy— just as the rhetoric of salvation drowned out the noise generated by the persecution of witches and their anguished cries of protest. It is a heartless hypocrisy to pretend that physicians, psychiatrists or normal laymen for that matter really care about the welfare of the mentally ill in general, or the homosexual in particular. If they did, they would stop torturing him while claiming to help him (Szasz, 1970: 168).

As alluded to by Szasz, the characterization of individuals or groups as deviant may lead not only to their marginalization, but to their stigmatization as well. It has been said that stigmatization

is essentially a relational construct; a stigmatized person must be marked or labeled as deviating from a social standard or norm, and the label must be socially constructed as negatively valued. An attributional component is inherent in most formulations of the stigma construct; the mark is regarded as the result or manifestation of a personal attribute, disposition, or trait. In other words, the stigmatized individual is perceived as guilty in some way for having caused or maintained their "marked" condition, even when no evidence for their culpability is readily apparent (Luchetta, 1999: 2).

Many times, these attributions and the associated stigmatization are premised on stereotypes. Those who are stigmatized

are pejoratively regarded by the broader society and [are] devalued, shunned or otherwise lessened in their life chances and in access to the humanizing benefit of free and unfettered social intercourse (Alonzo and Reynolds, 1995: 304).

Various international guidelines recognize the risk of stigmatization and marginalization that may result or be associated with participation in health-related research. The *International Guidelines for Biomedical Research Involving Human Subjects* (Council for International Organizations of Medical Sciences, 2002) notes in the commentary to Guideline 8, which addresses the benefits and risks of study participation, that

research in certain fields, such as epidemiology, genetics, or sociology, may present risks to the interests of communities, societies, or racially or ethnically defined groups. Information might be published that could stigmatize a group or expose its members to discrimination. Such information, for example, could indicate, rightly or wrongly, that the group has a higher than average prevalence of alcoholism, mental illness or sexually transmitted disease, or is particularly susceptible to certain genetic disorders. Plans to conduct such research should be sensitive to such consideration, to the need to maintain confidentiality during and after the study, and for the need to publish the resulting data in a manner that is respectful of the interests of all concerned, or in certain circumstances not to publish them. The ethical review committee should ensure that the interests of all concerned are given due consideration; often it will be advisable to have individual consent supplemented by community consultation.

Guidelines 19 and 21 of the *International Guidelines for the Ethical Review of Epidemiological Studies* (Council for International Organizations of Medical Sciences, 1991) also caution investigators to be aware of this potential risk and to protect research participants from such risk to the extent possible. Guideline 19 provides that "ethical review must always assess the risk of subjects or groups suffering stigmatization, prejudice, loss of prestige or self-esteem, or economic loss as a result of taking part in a study . . . ," while Guideline 21 notes that

Epidemiological studies may inadvertently expose groups as well as individuals to harm, such as economic loss, stigmatization, blame, or withdrawal of services. Investigators who find sensitive information that may put a group at risk of adverse criticism or treatment should be discreet in communicating and explaining their findings. When the location or circumstances of a study are important to understanding the results, the investigators will explain by what means they propose to protect the group from harm or disadvantage; such means include provisions for confidentiality and the use of language that does not imply moral criticism of subjects' behaviour.

The duty of the researcher to be cognizant of and to minimize such risks to the research participants arises from the ethical principles of beneficence and nonmaleficence. *Beneficence* refers to the "ethical obligation to maximize possible benefits and to minimize possible harms and wrongs," while the principle of *nonmaleficence* counsels researchers to protect participants from avoidable harms (Council for International Organizations of Medical Sciences, 1991).

Summary

It is critical that researchers consider the larger ethical, social, and political implications of their categorization of populations and research participants. Efforts must be made to reduce the likelihood that these categorizations, which may be formulated with the best of intentions to improve health, will result instead in the reinforcement of stereotypes and the marginalization and/or devaluation of specific groups.

References

Alonzo, A.A., Reynolds, N.R. (1995). Stigma, HIV and AIDS: An exploration and elaboration of a stigma trajectory. *Social Science and Medicine, 41(3)*, 303–315.

American Psychiatric Association. (1968). *Diagnostic and Statistical Manual, DSM-II.* Washington, D.C.: Author.

Bayer, R. (1981). *Homosexuality and American Psychiatry: The Politics of Diagnosis*. New York: Basic Books, Inc.

Bell, R.B. (1971). *Social Deviance*. Homewood, Illinois: Dorsey.

Ben-Yehuda, N. (1990). *The Politics and Morality of Deviance: Moral Panics, Drug Abuse, Deviant Science, and Diverse Stigmatization*. Albany, New York: State University of New York Press.

Comstock, G.D. (1991). *Violence against Lesbians and Gay Men*. New York: Columbia University Press.

Cullen, F.T., Cullen, J.B. (1978). *Toward a Paradigm of Labeling Theory*. Lincoln, Nebraska: University of Nebraska.

Erikson, K.T. (1962). Notes on the sociology of deviance. *Social Problems, 9*, 307–314.

Epstein, J. (1990). Either/or—neither/both: Sexual ambiguity and the ideology of gender. *Genders* 7: 99–142.

Freire, P. (1970). *Pedagogy of the Oppressed*. (Trans. M.B. Ramos). New York: Continuum.

Gibson, M., Meem, D.T. (Eds.). (2002). *Femme/Butch: New Considerations of the Way We Want to Go*. Binghamton, New York: Harrington Park Press.

Healey, D. (2001). *Homosexual Desire in Revolutionary Russia: The Regulation of Sexual and Gender Dissent*. Chicago, Illinois: University of Chicago Press.

Jenkins, R. (2003). Rethinking ethnicity: Identity, categorization, and power. In J. Stone, R. Dennis (Eds.), *Race and Ethnicity: Comparative and Theoretical Approaches* (pp. 58–71). Malden, Massachusetts: Blackwell Publishing.

Kitsuse, J.L. (1962). Societal reaction to deviant behavior: Problems of theory and method. *Social Problems* 9: 247–256.

Kittrie, N. (1972). *The Right to Be Different*. Baltimore, Maryland: Johns Hopkins University Press.

Luchetta, Y. (1999). Relationships between homophobia, HIV/AIDS stigma, and HIV/AIDS knowledge. In L. Pardie, T. Luchetta (Eds.), *The Construction of Attitudes Towards Lesbians and Gay Men* (pp. 1–18). Binghamton, New York: Harrington Park Press.

Mason, A., Palmer, A. (1996). *Queer Bashing: A National Survey of Hate Crimes against Lesbians and Gay Men*. London: Stonewall.

Stoller, R.J. (1991). *Pain and Passion: A Psychoanalyst Explores the World of S&M*. New York: Plenum Press.

Stone, D.A. (1988). *Policy Paradox and Political Reason*. Boston, Massachusetts: Little, Brown.

Stone, J. (2003). Max Weber on race, ethnicity, and nationalism. In J. Stone, R. Dennis (Eds.), *Race and Ethnicity: Comparative and Theoretical Approaches* (pp. 28–42). Malden, Massachusetts: Blackwell Publishing.

Szasz, T. (1970). *The Manufacture of Madness*. New York: Delta Books.

Tucker, M. (1990). Director's forward. In R. Ferguson, M. Gever, T.T. Minh-ha, C. West (Eds.), *Out There: Marginalization and Contemporary Cultures* (pp. 7–8). New York: The New Museum of Contemporary Art/MIT Press.

Wright, L. (1997). *The Bear Book: Readings in the History and Evolution of a Gay Male Subculture*. Binghamton, New York: Harrington Park Press.

Yanow, D. (2003). *Constructing "Race" and "Ethnicity" in America: Category-Making in Public Policy and Administration*. Armonk, New York: M.E. Sharpe.

2
Methodological Considerations

The selection of instruments for use in a particular study or the construction of new instruments to assess ethnicity, race, gender, sex, and related constructs requires a consideration of various methodological issues, in addition to the context in which these tools are to be developed and the ethical implications of the categories once they have been developed. Issues to be considered prior to deciding which of existing instruments to use or whether and how to construct a new instrument include the focus of the research question, the format to be used to collect the data, and how the population of interest is to be sampled. The selection of an instrument for use, or the development of a new instrument, also requires attention to the instrument's validity, reliability, and the possibility of misclassification associated with its use (McDowell and Newell, 1996). A basic understanding of these issues is important in order to better evaluate the literature that exists with regard to the constructs that are the focus of this text. This is not, however, a comprehensive discussion of these issues, which can be the focus of entire books themselves, and the reader is urged to consult the sources listed at the end of this chapter for additional guidance.

Framing the Research Question and the Research

How a research question is framed and the design of the study that will be undertaken for its investigation are critical issues to be resolved prior to identifying the instruments to be used or whether and how to develop a new instrument for the assessment of any of the constructs discussed in this text. Issues requiring consideration include the following.

(1) The time period of interest. Because one's self-identity may change over time with respect to ethnicity, race, sexual orientation, and related constructs, it is important to determine at what point in time these are to be assessed. For instance, does the research question demand an understanding of how an individual currently self-identifies? This might be relevant, for instance, in studies assessing current patient satisfaction with health care. Or, does the study focus on the impact of stigmatization on one's health status over time? In this case, it may be important

to assess the individual's identity over time and/or how an individual is perceived by others in terms of his or her race, ethnicity, sexual orientation, etc.

This is an important consideration even in instances in which the researcher has decided to rely on pre-formulated categories for the classification of the research participants. For instance, the manner in which the federal government has defined various ethnicities and races has changed over time. (See chapter 3.) A study that spans time periods that use different classification systems may find that the choices provided to respondents at the initiation of the study period may no longer be in use towards the end, and researchers may have to reconcile responses to the newer categories.

(2) The focus of the research question. The concepts of race, ethnicity, sex, gender, sexual orientation and related concepts are multidimensional. As an example, depending upon the focus of the research, a determination of ethnicity may require an assessment of the ethnicity of an individual's parents and grandparents in addition to a consideration of the origin of the individual research participant. A sexual history that focuses on the number and sex of one's sexual partners may be sufficient to answer a question focusing on the sex of one's sexual partners, but it may not be adequate to determine an individual's sexual orientation, which is a function of emotional attraction, physical attraction, sexual fantasies, self-definition, and opportunity.

These characteristics are also subject to identification not only by the individual who may be a participant in the research, but also by the observer as well. For instance, an individual may self-identify his or her race (suspending, for the moment, a discussion as to whether race exists), but an individual's race is also subject to the perception of the observer who, on the basis of criteria that he or she as somehow developed, will make a judgment regarding the individual's race. Consequently, it is important to consider in framing the research question whether participants' self-identity as to race, ethnicity, sexual orientation, gender, etc. is important or whether it is the perception of specified observers that is critical. For instance, how an individual identifies him- or herself with respect to race may not be as important as how the individual is viewed by others, if the focus of the study is an exploration of the effects of political marginalization.

Selecting the Sample

How the study sample is selected and the size of the sample are critical issues. A biased sample may lead to erroneous conclusions and an inadequate sample will not have sufficient statistical power to detect the hypothesized effect. This section very briefly reviews issues related to sampling. The issue is a complex one, and readers are referred to other texts for an in-depth exploration of the topic (Cochran, 1977; Kish, 1965; Levy and Lemeshow, 1980).

The sampling procedure is framed around the sampling unit. In many cases, this will be the individual, but it can be a family or household, or area of a community. The sample that will be constructed consists of the sampling units that have been selected from among those that are eligible for inclusion in the study (Kelsey, Thomson, and Evans, 1986). For example, if an investigator wished to know the proportion of households of a particular ethnic group had health insurance, the sample would consist of a portion of those households where a designated member was of that ethnicity.

The sampling frame refers to the list of the population from which the sample will be drawn. In some cases, this is unknown and unknowable. For instance, a study focusing on the experience of homophobia by gay and lesbian individuals would have a difficult, if not impossible, task to construct a sampling frame, since it would not be possible to know of every individual who self-identified as gay or lesbian, since many may not wish to acknowledge their orientation publicly.

In instances in which it would be difficult to locate and recruit study participants due to the nature of the research, investigators often rely on a convenience sample comprised of volunteers. This strategy, however, can introduce bias into the selection process. Snowball sampling, in which already-recruited participants identify other individuals as potential participants, permits investigators to more easily locate and recruit "hidden" individuals, but may also introduce selection bias because the individuals recruited through respondents are more likely to be like the respondents.

Probability sampling is advisable when it is feasible, in order to reduce the possibility of selection bias. There are four basic designs for probability sampling: simple random sampling, systematic sampling, stratified sampling, and cluster sampling.

Simple random sampling requires knowledge of the complete sampling frame in advance (Kelsey, Thompson, and Evans, 1986). This strategy means that each sampling unit in the population has an equal chance of being selected for participation. This method does not require advance knowledge of the population itself, but may be very inefficient.

Systematic sampling refers to the selection of sampling unit, such as individuals or households, at regularly spaced intervals within the sampling frame, such as every third household. This method has several advantages in that it does not require advance knowledge of the sampling frame, as it can be constructed as the process progresses and is generally relatively simple to implement.

Stratified sampling requires the division of the population into strata and a sample is selected from each such strata. This process is significantly more complex than the other strategies, but offers increased precision and may facilitate the inclusion of specific groups of persons.

Like stratified sampling, cluster sampling divides the sample into groups, such as clusters of homes. A sample is then taken of these clusters for inclusion in the study or, alternatively, a subsample of these sample clusters is utilized. As an example, an investigator wishing to study the prevalence of violence in public housing projects might divide all such projects into clusters by geographic area and then take a sample of these clusters. The households within these clusters could then be queried about the violence in the public housing projects.

Data Collection

Numerous strategies can be used to collect race/ethnicity/sexual orientation data including self-administered questionnaires and surveys, telephone interviews, and face-to-face interviews. Questions can be open-ended, or respondents can be presented with a pre-formulated listing of acceptable responses. Or, researchers may decide to rely on secondary databases and must necessarily, then, utilize the categories embedded in those databases. Depending upon the source of the database, respondents may have had to select their responses from a pre-formulated list, or the categorization of the individual may have been accomplished by an interviewer. The strategies that are selected have implications for the response that will be obtained. These various approaches are compared below.

Self-Completed Instruments versus Interviews

There are advantages and disadvantages associated with either strategy of having respondents complete instruments on their own, or conducting telephone or in-person interviews with respondents.

Self-completed instruments, whether with pencil and paper or through the use of a computer, have the potential to obtain more accurate responses from participants for several reasons. First, because the individual does not have to interact with anyone in giving the response, he or she may be more willing and comfortable to divulge particularly sensitive or embarrassing information in this manner. Computer-assisted self-interviewing (CASI), which permits respondents to type their answers on a computer keyboard in response to items on the computer screen, may be particularly helpful (Camburn and Cynamon, 1993; O'Reilly, Hubbard, Lessler, Biemer, and Turner, 1994). Second, the individual may feel less time pressure to complete the instrument because they are not facing or speaking with anyone directly. As a result, their answers may be more thoughtful.

However, there are several problems associated with self-completed instruments. Individuals may not be able to read or read well and may be embarrassed to disclose this. If this is the situation, they may be tempted to circle any response or write in any number just to complete the form. Unless the instruments are reviewed immediately by someone with the individual still there, it is also possible that individuals may have inadvertently missed items and the instrument remains incomplete. In some cases, depending upon the study design and/or the study population, it may be difficult to relocate or contact the respondent to obtain the missing data. Additionally, self-completed instruments are generally not appropriate for questions that are complex or open-ended and would require lengthier responses (Aday, 1996).

In-person or telephone interviews offer several advantages in that they allow investigators to complete an instrument with a participant, so the participant's ability to read may not be relevant and it is less likely that items contained in the instruments will be inadvertently missed. However, there may be an increased likelihood that answers will be inaccurate of the questions are felt to be embarrassing or stigmatizing. With phone interviews, particularly if there has not already been a relationship established with the study, there is a greater chance that the prospective participant will simply hang-up or that they will screen calls and not answer (Aday, 1996).

Respondent Self-identification versus Observer Identification

A decision as to who should categorize the research respondent is going to depend to a great extent on the focus of the research question: is it the individual's self-identity that is at issue or the perceptions of others that are most relevant?

By allowing respondents to self-classify with respect to any of the variables of interest discussed in this text, the researcher will be better able to understand definitions and distinctions internal to the community of interest. For example, in a study conducted by Carballo-Diéguez and Dolezal (1994) in which they allowed respondents to self-identify with respect to sexual orientation, they found that among Latino men who have sex with men (MSM) who had had at least one male partner during the previous year, 20% self-identified as bisexual or *hombres modernos* (modern men), 10% self-identified as heterosexual, 65% self-identified as gay, and 4% self-identified as drag queens; 80% of those self-identifying as bisexual had had sex with a woman during the previous year, in comparison with 63% of the men self-identifying as heterosexual; and almost three-fifths of the men self-identifying as gay had had sexual relations with a woman; 8% had had sex with a woman during the previous year. Had they presented respondents with a preformulated list from which to select their sexual orientation, they would not have been able to understand the distinctions made within this community that are relevant to both risk behaviors and prevention interventions.

Allowing respondents to self-identify may then provide the researcher with additional flexibility in the development of the categories to be utilized in the study. A large number of categories resulting from respondent self-definition can be collapsed into fewer categories to increase statistical power.

Participant self-identification may, however, create difficulties for the researcher as well as providing these advantages. The terms selected by respondents to self-identify may not be comparable to categories then in use in the literature, making comparison across research studies difficult. Additionally, respondents may differ in the characteristics they choose as a basis for self-identification. For instance, in asking respondents to describe their ethnicity, some research participants may focus on their country of origin, some on their religion, some on the culture of their parents or grandparents, etc. The researcher may not be aware of the varying criteria used and may have difficulty reframing the responses.

Identification based on observer perception has the advantage of consistent application of pre-specified criteria. However, as described in chapter 3, there is often considerable variance between observer perception of identity and an individual's self-definition. The importance of any resulting difference necessarily depends on the focus of the research.

Pre-formulated Lists versus Open-Ended Questioning

The issue of whether to use pre-formulated lists or open-ended questioning is related to the issue of respondent versus observer identification of an individual. In general, researchers who rely on observer classification of participants with respect to race or ethnicity often work from a pre-formulated list, while the use of open-ended questioning is more frequently employed when relying on participant self-identification.

Pre-formulated lists offer numerous advantages to the researcher. Because there is a predetermined number of categories, analysis may be simpler and, particularly with smaller sample sizes, use of a small number of categories for any particular construct may enhance statistical power. However, reliance on pre-formulated lists presents difficulties if the levels of a variable are overlapping or if they do not consider all possible responses. (See discussion regarding the interpretation of categories, below.)

Regardless of whether one ultimately decides to utilize a pre-formulated list of categories from which to select a response or to have participants answer open-ended questions, the ordering of the questions may be critical. Various approaches are available to order questions. The ordering may be done

- Temporally, from earlier events to more recent events or from more recent events to events occurring in the more distant past
- According to complexity, from simpler topics or concepts to ones that involve increasing complexity
- According to themes, so that questions pertaining to the same theme are grouped together
- By level of abstraction, so that the most concrete items are grouped together and the most abstract are grouped together
- According to level of sensitivity, so that the items that require the greatest level of personal disclosure or focus on the most sensitive topics follow those that are the least sensitive (Schensul, Schensul, and LeCompte, 1999).

Using Scales

There are three primary forms of scales that are often utilized in health research: the Likert, Guttman, and Thurstone Equal-Appearing Interval Scales. Readers are referred to other sources for a more in-depth discussion regarding the construction of scales (Aday, 1996; Spector, 1992).

A Likert scale utilizes an ordinal response scale which allows the respondent to indicate his or her level of agreement of disagreement with a particular item. Five categories of agreement/disagreement are generally used: strongly agree, agree, uncertain or neutral, disagree, strongly disagree. A score is assigned to each such level and the scores are summed across all items to yield a summary score. The Adolescent Survey of Black Life (Table 7 in chapter 6) illustrates the use of a Likert scale.

In contrast, a Guttman scale is premised on the idea that there is a hierarchy in attitudes or perceptions and this hierarchy can be utilized to construct the scale. Positive responses to each item within a hierarchy are totaled to yield a total score (Aday, 1996).

The construction of a Thurstone Equal-Appearing Interval Scale is based on the ratings of items by a selected group of judges as to the extent to which they reflect a negative or positive attitude toward the issue in question. The judges are asked to place these items along an 11-point scale, ranging from most unfavorable to most favorable. The overall degree of favorableness of a particular items is determined by the median value of all of the judges with respect to that particular item. The items that have the least agreement among the judges re eliminated and the remaining ones are incorporated into a questionnaire (Aday, 1996).

Several factors should be considered in deciding whether to construct a new scale for a particular study or to use an existing one. The use of an existing scale may be preferable if it has been shown to have a high degree of reliability and validity and has been tested in the same or similar population as the study population to be assessed. The investigator should also consider whether it is available in the language used by the study population.

Validity

Four types of validity will be discussed here: content validity, criterion validity, construct validity, and factorial validity. *Content validity* refers to the comprehensiveness of the questions asked and whether they adequately reflect the intended goals. For instance, in designing an instrument to assess gender role, the investigator must ensure that all of the questions are relevant to the concept of gender role and that all salient aspects of gender role are covered by the questions. One way to assess the content validity of a proposed instrument is to ask other professionals familiar with the content area to review the items. Focus groups can be conducted with individuals who are representative of the groups with which the instrument is to be used, in order to get their feedback and suggestions to improve both the content of the instrument and the wording of its items. It may be difficult, however, to establish definitively that all of the items included in the instrument reflect all relevant items (Seiler, 1973).

In contrast, the term *criterion validity* refers to the extent to which an instrument correlates with another "gold standard" instrument designed to assess the same factor(s). The term criterion validity can be used with respect to particular items of an instrument or the instrument as a whole. Unfortunately, no instrument exists that is considered the gold standard for the assessment of many of the themes discussed in this text. Indeed, given the diversity that exists within and between communities, it is difficult to conceive of such a gold standard.

The *criterion validity* of an instrument can be assessed by calculating its sensitivity and specificity. *Sensitivity* refers to the proportion of individuals with a particular characteristic who are correctly classified as having that characteristic.

The question then becomes how to determine what the correct classification is. Since there is no instrument that is considered the gold standard, the classification of items by the newly constructed instrument cannot be assessed against the gold standard. One way to accomplish this comparison and assess sensitivity, however, might be to compare the results of the new instrument against individuals' self-classification. Conversely, the term *specificity* is the proportion of individuals without a specific characteristic who are correctly assessed by the instrument as being without that characteristic. The sensitivity and specificity of an instrument can be combined to give a single measure of accuracy. (For a discussion of how to calculate sensitivity, specificity, and accuracy, see McDowell and Newell, 1996; Morgenstern, 1996).

Construct validity requires that a conceptual definition of the construct be formulated, including the components of that concept. There is no perfect way to assess construct validity. Instead, construct validity may be suggested by the extent to which the results produced by the newly designed instrument correlate or do not correlate with other assessment instruments designed to measure the same constructs. For example, a high degree of correlation between the findings of a newly designed instrument to assess gender role and a pre-existing instrument used to assess the same construct would suggest that the new instrument displays *convergent validity*, said to be equivalent to assessing sensitivity (McDowell and Newell, 1996). If the new instrument does not correlate well with other instruments designed to assess different themes, it can be said that it displays *divergent validity*. However, it is unclear how high a level of correlation is required to say that there is adequate correlation (McDowell and Newell, 1996).

Factor analysis is often used to examine the conceptual structure of an instrument by assessing how well the items of the instrument fall into expected groupings. Using again the example of an instrument designed to measure gender role across various contexts, we might use factor analysis to determine whether the questions fall into two or more distinct groups such as masculinity and femininity. These groupings should be homogenous and unrelated to each other. (For a discussion of the difficulties associated with such a distinction, see chapter 3.)

The appropriate use of factor analysis requires that the variables be assessed using an interval-level scale (McDowell and Newell, 1996); reliance on interval-level scales may be somewhat rare in the context of assessing the constructs discussed in this text. Where this approach is used, though, it is important that there be at least five times the number of respondents in the sample than there are variables to be used in the analysis (McDowell and Newell, 1996). However, many journal articles may indicate that factor analysis was used to evaluate the content validity of instruments that utilize categorical responses, such as "never," "sometimes," "frequently," "always."

Reliability

In addition to assessing the validity of an instrument, it is important to determine its reliability. *Reliability* refers to the consistency of a measurement across time, respondents, and/or observers. Reliability is said to consist of two components: the true value of the measurement and a degree of error in the measurement that is obtained. Reliability is concerned with that portion of the measurement error that is random; the portion that is not random, or systematic, is referred to as bias. (Bias is discussed below in the context of misclassification.) Random error may occur for any number of reasons including interviewer fatigue, carelessness, and/or interviewee fatigue.

Inter-rater agreement or reliability refers to the extent to which different raters assess the respondent similarly. Inter-rater reliability for nominal or categorical data, such as categories of sexual orientation or ethnicity, can be reported using the Kappa coefficient. The kappa coefficient is obtained by constructing a table that indicates the proportion of agreement between the two raters. A weighted kappa formula is useful in discriminating between minor and major discrepancies between raters (Streiner and Norman, 1989).

Intra-rater reliability or test-retest reliability pertains to the assessment of a respondent by the same rater, and the extent to which a second assessment is consistent with the first, respectively. It has been recommended that the time interval between the assessments be brief in order to reduce the risk that an instrument will erroneously appear to be unreliable when it is actually detecting changes that have occurred between the assessments (McDowell and Newell, 1996). However, if the successive administrations of the instrument are spaced closely in time, the rater and/or the respondent may remember the answers to the previously administered assessment and this may influence the results of the subsequent assessment.

Various strategies have been formulated in an attempt to reduce these possibilities. The subsequent assessment may utilize an instrument that is parallel to the first, but that is not the same. The assessment of reliability in this situation would focus on the level of correlation between the two results. Alternatively, two equivalent but not identical versions of the same test can be merged into a single instrument to be utilized in a single session. Reliability is assessed by determining the comparability of the results if the measurement had been divided into two component versions (McDowell and Newell, 1996). This can be done by correlating odd- and even-numbered questions or by estimating correlations between all possible pairs of items. A greater level of correlation among the items will facilitate the correlation of two equivalent versions.

It should be noted that a higher level of internal consistency will produce greater test-retest reliability. Cronbach's alpha is often utilized to assess internal consistency. An unsatisfactory score for internal consistency can sometimes be improved by deleting items from the instrument that do not correlate highly with other items. However, the deletion of items that are critical to the construct(s) under evaluation may threaten the content validity of the instrument.

Misclassification

Misclassification, which is a form of information bias, occurs when the exposure or outcome status of a study participant is erroneously classified. Where the error depends on the value of other variables, the misclassification is said to be differential; nondifferential misclassification occurs when the classification error is not dependent on the values of other variables (Rothman and Greenland, 1998).

Assume, for instance, that an investigator wishes to evaluate the relationship between race/ethnicity and risk of lung cancer. The nondifferential misclassification of race or ethnicity could potentially mask any association that might exist and, if severe enough, could even reverse the direction of the association.

Similarities between some selection biases and misclassification bias are apparent. For instance, assume that an investigator wishes to oversample study participants from a particular ethnic group. Assume further that a portion of those individuals are erroneously classified as members of a different ethnic group and are considered eligible or ineligible for study participation on the basis of this erroneous classification. This is an example of selection bias. The information that will be derived from their participation in the study may suffer from information bias due to the continuing misclassification of those individuals who have been enrolled into the study on the basis of this erroneous classification.

The constructs that are the focus of this text, such as sex and ethnicity, are often considered to be confounding variables where they are associated with both the disease and the exposure under investigation, they are associated with the exposure among the source population for cases, and they are not on the causal pathway between the exposure and the disease. The nondifferential misclassification of a confounding variable will reduce the extent to which the confounding may be controlled. As a consequence, bias may occur either towards or away from the null value, depending upon the direction of the confounding. The results can be especially misleading if there is a weak association between the exposure and the disease of interest and the confounding is strong (Rothman and Greenland, 1998).

Interpreting Categories

The construction of categories often requires interpretation. Yanow (2003) has identified six features: (1) category errors, (2) a defining point of view, (3) tacit knowledge, (4) marking, (5), occluded features and silences, and (6) situated, local knowledge and change. The construction of categories implies, first, that everything that can be encompassed within a category actually is and, second, that there is no overlap in these characteristics across the named categories (Yanow, 2003). Difficulties occur when items do not fall within any of the named categories or when their characteristics permit their classification into more than one of the existing categories. As an example, true hermaphrodites may be considered to be of both male and female sexes or of neither male nor female sex. (See chapter 4 for further discussion regarding categories of sex.)

In discussing "a defining point of view," Yanow (2003) is referring to the manner in which categories are constructed, through the shared logic of a group of people about what characteristics are most salient to the construction of categories. The logic that underlies this shared category-making is often tacit, and may not appear logical to members of other groups ("tacit knowledge"). For instance, the United

States until recently has utilized a "one drop rule," whereby any indication of black ancestry indicated that an individual was racially black. This system might seem less than logical to individuals from societies in which skin color is viewed on a continuum, extending from very light to very dark. Tacit knowledge also operates where deviations from the norm ("marked cases") are assessed against those that are considered prototypical. What is considered deviant, or "marked," may not be obvious to those outside of the group constructing the category on the basis of tacit knowledge. The classification of homosexuality as deviant behavior is premised on a view of what is normal sexual behavior that is not universally shared.

A focus on specific features in the construction of categories may deflect attention from other, critical features, thereby occluding or obscuring them. A focus on skin color to explain health disparities, for instance, may deflect attention from issues that may be equally important or even more important to an understanding of existing disparities, such as differences in socioeconomic status or inability to access care due to lack of medical insurance.

Categories are not fixed; they are situated in local knowledge and, therefore, may change over time and reflect changes in local knowledge over time. Homosexuality was once categorized by the American Psychiatric Association as a mental illness, but is no longer included as such in its nosology. (See chapter 4.) Intersexuality continues to be viewed, in general, as an abnormal condition, but this understanding is being challenged in significant ways and it is possible that intersex conditions may, in the future, be considered as yet another reflection of biological diversity, rather than a condition requiring a cure. (See chapter 3). If this were to occur, the categorization of intersexuality as a medical condition in need of treatment would no longer be valid.

Summary

This chapter has explored the meaning of "category" and the various ethical implications and methodological complexities associated with the construction of categories. It is critical that researchers be cognizant of intragroup classifications in formulating categories to be used in their research and the risks that participants may face as a result of being associated with those categories. Researchers must also consider the validity and reliability of the measures used to delineate between various categories, the implications of misclassification, and the complexities involved in interpreting the resulting findings.

References

Aday, L. (1996). *Designing and Conducting Health Surveys*, 2nd ed. San Francisco, California: Jossey-Bass Publishers.

Carballo-Diéguez, A., Dolezal, C. (1994). Contrasting types of Puerto Rican men who have sex with men (MSM). *Journal of Psychology and Human Sexuality* 6(4): 41–67.

Cochran, W.G. (1977). *Sampling Techniques*. New York: Wiley.

Kelsey, J.L., Thomson, W.D., Evans, A.S. (1986). *Methods in Observational Epidemiology*. New York: Oxford University Press.

Kish, L. (1965). *Survey Sampling*. New York: Wiley.

Levy, P.S., Lemeshow, S. (1980). *Sampling for Health Professionals*. Belmont, California: Lifetime Learning Publications.

McDowell, I., Newell, C. (1996). *Measuring Health: A Guide to Rating Scales and Questionnaires,* 2nd ed. New York: Oxford University Press.

Morgenstern, H. (1996). *Course Materials, Part II: Class Notes for Epidemiologic Methods, Epidemiology 201B*, University of California Los Angeles.

Rothman, K.J., Greenland, S. (1998). *Modern Epidemiology*, 2nd ed. Philadelphia, Pennsylvania: Lippincott-Raven Publishers.

Schensul, S.L., Schensul, J.J., LeCompte, M.D. (1999). *Essential Ethnographic Methods: Observations, Interviews, and Questionnaires*. Walnut Creek, California: AltaMira Press.

Seiler, L.H. (1973). The 22-item scale used in field studies of mental illness: A question of method, a question of substance, and a question of theory. *Journal of Health and Social Behavior* 14: 252–264.

Spector, P.E. (1992). *Summated Rating Scale Construction: An Introduction*. Thousand Oaks, California: Sage.

Streiner, D.L., Norman, G.R. (1989). *Health Measurement Scales: A Practical Guide to Their Development and Use*. New York: Oxford University Press.

Yanow, D. (2003). *Constructing "Race" and "Ethnicity" in America: Category-Making in Public Policy and Administration*. Armonk, New York: M.E. Sharpe.

Part II
Constructs: Their Definition and Use

3
Defining Race, Ethnicity, and Related Constructs

Race

Science appears to have focused on the concept of race among human beings through the work of the biological taxonomist Carolus Linnaeus who, in 1735, classified human beings into four categories based upon their skin color: red, yellow, white, and black (Ehrlich and Feldman, 1977). Linnaeus further distinguished between the races based upon an amalgam of characteristics that he believed were associated with each. Whites, for instance, were said to be innovative, in contrast to blacks, who were deemed to be lazy and careless. Other scholars have credited Johann Friedrich Blumenbach, who in 1795 divided mankind into Caucasian, Mongolian, Ethiopian, American, and Malayan races, for the emergence of racial classification in western Europe and the United States (Sanjek, 1994). Regardless of who deserves such credit, from thenceforth, race would be associated with ascribed mental and moral traits.

The concept of race has since been used to explain perceived differences in appearance and in behavior across individuals and groups (Gaines, 1994). A variety of other criteria has also been used to define race, including region or geographical area of origin (King and Stansfield, 1990), nationality (Taylor, 1988), language, and religion (Gaines, 1994). These distinctions have provided the basis for various suppositions about race in the United States: that there exists a fixed number of races (Campbell, 1981; Becker and Landav, 1992; Segen, 1992), some of which are superior to others and each of which is characterized by distinct physical, mental or behavioral attributes that are reproduced over time (Boas, 1940; Gould, 1981; Montagu, 1964a).

The absence of conceptual clarity in defining "race" is evident from the variation in definition and classification over time, place, and purpose of designation (Osborne and Feit, 1992; Gaines, 1994; LaVeist, 1994). The United States alone has used a multitude of terms and definitions in an attempt to distinguish those who are white from those who are not (Davis, 1991). As an example, the censuses of 1840, 1850, and 1860 counted mulattoes, but did not explain what the term signified. The 1870 and 1880 censuses defined mulattoes as "quadroons, octoroons, and all persons having any perceptible trace of African blood" (Davis,

1991). The 1890 census required that enumerators record the exact proportion of "African blood," whereas the 1900 census required that "pure Negroes" be distinguished from mulattoes, who were then-defined as persons "with some trace of black blood" (Davis, 1991).

As of the 1930 census, "black" was defined as any individual with any black blood. In 1960, the basis for enumeration changed again, this time to permit the head of the household, rather than the enumerator, to identify the race of the household members (Davis, 1991). Prior to 1989, the assignment of race on birth certificates was to indicate "white" only if both parents were considered white (LaVeist, 1994), in accordance with the previously existing "one drop rule," whereby individuals with any observable black ancestry were to be defined as black (Stone and Dennis, 2003). Accordingly, a child born to one black parent and one white parent would have been designated at birth as a mulatto if born in 1900, but as a black if born in 1930. The 1990 census requested that respondents report their racial classification as the one with which they most closely identified. However, no definition of race was provided, resulting in confusion and "misreporting" (McKenney and Bennett, 1994).

Confusion is also evident in the classification over time of Hispanics in the United States. In 1930, those of Mexican-origin who were not "definitely White, Negro, Indian, Chinese, or Japanese" were classified for census purposes as Mexican (Martin, DeMaio, and Campanelli, 1990). By 1960, Mexicans, Puerto Ricans, and "Others of Latin descent" were deemed to be White unless they were determined by observation to be Negro, Indian, "or some other race." In 1980, Hispanics were able to self-identify as black, white, or other (Martin et al., 1990).

In order to standardize the categories and definitions used by federal agencies to collect data pertaining to race, the federal Office of Management and Budget formulated what eventually came to be known as OMB Statistical Policy Directive No. 15, "Race and Ethnic Standards for Federal Statistics and Administrative Reporting." The standards embodied in this document were to be utilized by all federal agencies collecting data pertaining to race and/or ethnicity on or after January 1, 1980 (Yanow, 2003). However, as can be seen in Table 1 below, the categories and definitions established by this directive have been changed over time. For instance, in 1977, according to these definitions, a person born in Samoa would have been Asian or Pacific Islander for census purposes but, if born in 2000, would have been classified as Native Hawaiian or Other Pacific Islander.

Yanow (2003) has raised significant questions with respect to this schema that underscore the problematic and arbitrary nature of these categories. First, what are origins and how far back must one go to determine what they are? Second, in referring to "original peoples," how does one determine what or who they are and how far back in time must one go to determine this? Third, why are Blacks deemed to have their origins in racial groups, Hispanics in cultures or geographic origins, and others in original peoples? Finally, why is identification as American Indian or Alaska Native linked to tribal affiliation or community attachment, whereas this is not a requirement for identification in any other category?

TABLE 1. Comparison of categories and definitions for race and ethnicity developed by federal office of management and budget

Categories and definitions pursuant to 1977/1980 OMB directive no. 15	Categories and definitions pursuant to 1997 OMB directive no. 15
American Indian or Alaskan Native: A person having origins in any of the original peoples of North America, and who maintains cultural identification through tribal affiliation or community recognition	*American Indian or Alaska Native*: A person having origins in any of the original people of North and South America (including Central America and who maintains tribal affiliation or community attachment
Asian or Pacific Islander: A person having origins in any of the original peoples of the Far East, Southeast Asia, the Indian subcontinent or the Pacific Islands including, for example, China, India, Japan, Korea, the Philippine Islands, Samoa	*Asian*: A person having origins in any of the original peoples of the Far East, or the Indian subcontinent including, for example, Cambodia, China, India, Japan, Korea, Malaysia, Pakistan, the Philippine Islands, Thailand, and Vietnam
	Native Hawaiian or Other Pacific Islander: A person having origins in any of the original peoples of Hawaii, Guam, Samoa, or other Pacific Islands
Black: A person having origins in any of the black racial groups of Africa	*Black or African American*: A person having origins in any of the black racial groups of Africa. Terms such as "Haitian" or "Negro" can be used in addition to "Black or African American"
Hispanic: A person of Mexican, Puerto Rican, Cuban, Central or South American, or other Spanish culture or origin, regardless of race.	*Hispanic or Latino*: A person of Cuban, Mexican, Puerto Rican, South or Central American, or other Spanish culture or origin, regardless of race. The term "Spanish origin" can be used in addition to "Hispanic or Latino"
White: A person having origins in any of the original peoples of Europe, North Africa, or the Middle East	*White*: A person having origins in any of the original peoples of Europe, the Middle East, or North Africa

Classification of individuals as American Indian is particularly problematic. Even if an individual is recognized by his tribe as a member, he or she may not be considered an American Indian for various federal purposes unless he or she is able to demonstrate a sufficient quantum of "Indian blood" that is specified by federal regulations and tribal specification (Jaimes, 1994). In yet other circumstances, an individual may qualify for some federal entitlements through the production of a "Certificate with Degree of Indian Blood" issued by a regional agency of the Bureau of Indian Affairs, even if the tribal community in which they claim membership does not recognize them as a member according to the traditional system of kinship (Jaimes, 1990).

Designation of a person's race has varied by place as well. Indeed, in many countries, such as Brazil, Morocco, and Nicaragua, color consciousness is embodied in a process that is significantly more complex and multifaceted than the one drop rule was (Stone and Dennis, 2003). The black/mulatto child born in the

United States would be classified as a mulatto in Brazil, and further categorized by the degree of darkness or lightness of the skin color as a *preto* (black), *preto retinto* (dark black), *cabra* (slightly less black), *escuro* (lighter), *mulato esuro* (dark mulatto), *mulato claro* (light mulatto), *sarara, moreno, blanca de terra*, or *blanco* (LaVeist, 1994). Similarly, a "black" person in the United States would be classified in Cuba into one of various categories based upon both skin color and hair texture: *moro, indiano*, or *jabao* (Navarro, 1997). In South Africa, the term "black" encompasses individuals from India and those deemed to have mixed racial heritage (McNeil, 1998), while in the U.S., those from India are classified as Asian. In the West Indies, "Trinidad white" refers to individuals of mixed European and island parentage (Segal, 1991). Prior to 1989 in the United States, a child born to a "white" father and a Japanese mother would have been classified as Japanese on his or her birth certificate. In pre-1985 Japan, the same child would have been classified as white on the birth certificate (LaVeist, 1994).

The designation of a person's color in Nicaragua may be particularly complex. According to the widely recognized phenotypic system, individuals are classifiable as *blanco* (white), *moreno* (brown), or *negro* (black) (Lancaster, 2003). The term *blanco* is used to refer to individuals with primarily European ancestry. The category *moreno* includes the vast mestizo (Spanish-speaking, primarily indigenous) population, defined culturally and often characterized by brown hair and brown skin, while the term *negro* denotes those of African ancestry or individuals who are "indigenous" in appearance, whether further classified as Indio (Indian) or mestizo. In more polite usage, a different system of classification prevails: *chele*, or *rubio*, denotes those who are phenotypically blanco (with light hair and blue eyes, for example); *blanco* is now used to refer to phenotypical *morenos* (brown hair and brown skin), and the term *moreno* is used to designate those who would be *negro* under the phenotypic system. The pejorative usage of the terms delineates only two groups: *chele*, to refer to those with lighter hair and fairer skin tone, and *negro*, meaning those with darker skin and hair. These terms can be used pejoratively, as in *negro hijo de puta* (black son of a whore) or affectionately, as in the family nickname, *negrito* (little black one). Table 2, below, contrasts these three systems.

TABLE 2. Comparison of three approaches to color classification in Nicaragua

Characteristics	Phenotypic system	Polite usage	Pejorative and affectionate usage
Primarily European ancestry, white skin, blue eyes	*blanco*	*chele, rubio*	*chele*
Spanish-speaking indigenous population, mestizo, brown skin, hair, and eyes	*moreno*	*blanco*	*negro*
Black	*negro*	*moreno* (includes dark brown skin)	*negro* (referring to darker skin and darker hair)

Adapted from Lancaster, 2003.

Lancaster (2003: 109–110) has explained how this multifaceted approach is implemented in daily life:

Color discriminations there constitute themselves not so much as solid, permanent structures but as a series of discursive gestures that are contingent and contextual and whose motives are eminently logical and self-interested. The site of these distinctions knows no bounds; they operate equally within the self, the family, the neighborhood, and society at large. Indeed, this system exists always as a practice, never as a structure; there is no trace boundary, no race line, no stopping point where negotiation and discourse cease .... Not an absolute boundary at all, these color distinctions are best seen as a series of concentric circles, which are in fact power plays, emanating from a highly problematic ego who may win or lose depending on contingent factors.

The designation of race has varied even among the various states within the United States. As an example, "privileges of whites" were extended to a "quadroon" female by the Supreme Court of Ohio in 1831 due to "the difficulty of ... ascertaining the degree of duskiness which renders a person liable to such disabilities" (*Gray v. Ohio*, 1831). However, the California Supreme Court construed the word "white" to exclude "black, yellow, and all other colors .... The term 'black person' is to be construed as including everyone who is not of white blood" (*People v. Hall*, 1854).

The purpose or process of racial designation may also affect the ultimate classification of an individual. For example, a child's race on his or her birth certificate is designated by the infant's mother. At death, the assignment of race is often made by the funeral director in order to complete the death certificate. An individual classified as one race at birth by his or her parent may be classified as another race at death, suggesting that race is, indeed, in the eye of the beholder (Hahn, 1992). A study of almost 118,000 live births in North Carolina in 2002 found that mothers reported more than 600 different versions of race on their children's birth certificates (Buescher, Gizlice, and Jones-Vessey, 2005). The most common designations were white, black, Hispanic, Asian, and American Indian. Entries also included specific nationalities, such as Dominican and British; racial or nationality combinations, such as white/Mexican and Egyptian/Canadian; and some entries that could not be easily categorized, such as "Son of God." Because North Carolina vital records must be coded to a single racial group for the purpose of reporting to the National Center for Health Statistics, all text entries for race were required to be converted into one of 10 categories: white, black, Indian, Chinese, Japanese, Hawaiian, Filipino, Other Asian or Pacific Islander, Other Entries, and not reported. Specific rules exist for these conversions. As an example, if "Hawaiian" is reported together with any other race, the individual is to be coded as Hawaiian. In all other cases in which multiple races are reported, the individual is to be recorded as having the first race listed. These conversions procedures resulted in the significant discrepancies in identification between self-reports and NCHS coding results: 63.4% self-reported status as white, compared with NCHS coding of 72.7% as white; 23.0% self-reported black and 23.4% were coded as black for NCHS; 1.3% self-reported Indian, 1.4% Indian per NCHS coding; and 12.3% fell into other categories and combinations according to self-report, but only 2.4% did so according to NCHS coding procedures. Such discrepancies are troublesome because the resulting proportions may be utilized to assess the existence of health care disparities and these proportions differ depending upon how race is classified. For instance, using self-reported racial status, blacks were 2.42 times more likely than whites to receive late or no prenatal care. However, reliance on NCHS coding indicates that blacks are 1.94 times more likely than whites to receive late or no prenatal care(Buescher, Gizlice, and Jones-Vessey, 2005).

Another study of the National Center for Health Statistics found that 5.8% of the individuals who reported themselves as "black" were classified as "white" by the interviewer, while 32.3% of the self-reported Asians and 70% of the self-reported Native Americans were classified by the interviewer as either "white" or "black" (Massey, 1980). A comparison of administrative data with self-reported race and ethnicity among patients receiving services from the Veterans Administration indicated only a 60% rate of agreement between data sources. As an example of these discrepancies, it was found that African Americans were misclassified as white almost 5% of the time. Better agreement was noted for individuals who were less educated, young, and white, who were not living by themselves, and who made greater use of inpatient services (Kressin, Chang, Hendricks, and Kazis, 2003). A study examining the consistency between self-reported ethnicity recorded in Kaiser hospital admissions databases found significant disagreement in the recording of ethnicity for Hispanic and Native American patients (Gomez, Kelsey, Glaser, Lee, and Sidney, 2005). The Health Care Financing Administration has also noted misclassification in data collected about elderly Medicare enrollees (Lauderdale and Goldberg, 1996).

The meaning or significance that attaches to a particular designation may vary over time and place, as well. In Nicaragua, whiteness is a desired quality and how white or nonwhite an individual is, is relative to the context and those around him or her. Lancaster (2003: 107–108) has explained:

Where power and privilege are at stake, white implies might and right, as it were. When people employ the ambiguity of color terms to their own advantage, when they shift from one descriptive scale to another, and when they negotiate their own location within a system of contrasts, they are struggling over honor, to be sure, but they are no less struggling over privilege and power....

Whiteness thus serves as a kind of symbolic capital, empowering its claimant to make advantageous exchanges in a host of other symbolic and material realms.... Color terms constitute, symbolically, a series of representational strata; the people to whom they are applied experience, materially, differential life chances. Although not absolute, the correspondence of economic classes to the representational color scheme is by no means random. From a semiotic point of view, these color relations are ultimately power relations, and they constitute ... a substratum as much as a superstructure.

Another example is provided by an examination of the term "yellow race." In the United States, the use of this phrase to refer to Asians was pejorative. However, throughout much of Chinese history, the color yellow was associated with nobility and grandeur and to be of the yellow race was to be superior. Indeed, the Chinese writer Tan Caichang (1867–1900) wrote, "Yellow and white are wise, red and black are stupid; yellow and white are rulers, red and black are slaves; yellow and white are united, red and black are scattered" (Dikötter, 2003: 127). Primary schools in mainland China in 1920 taught as part of the curriculum:

Mankind is divided into five races. The yellow and white races are relatively strong and intelligent. Because the other races are feeble and stupid, they are being exterminated by the white race. This is so-called evolution... Among the contemporary races that could be called superior, there are only the yellow and the white races. China is the yellow race (Dikötter, 2003: 130, citing an original Chinese text).

Since the advent of AIDS, official discourse in China has depicted the disease as an evil from abroad, while popular discourse characterizes the epidemic as a threat against the pure blood of the Chinese people by the polluted blood of outsiders, implicitly merging concepts of race with the notion of national identity (Dikötter, 2003).

Too, one cannot assume that the designation of a group as delineated by those outside the group (etic) are the same as the categories that are constructed by members within that same group (emic) or that the categories, even if similar, hold the same meaning for those inside and outside of the group. For instance, Russell and colleagues (1992: 4–6) observed of African-Americans:

Traditionally, the color complex involved light-skinned Blacks' rejection of Blacks who were darker. Increasingly, however, the color complex shows up in the form of dark-skinned African Americans spurning their lighter-skinned brothers and sisters for not being Black enough. The complex even includes attitudes about hair texture, nose shape, and eye color. In short, the "color complex" is a psychological fixation about color and features that leads Blacks to discriminate against each other.... (Russell, Wilson, and Hall, 1992: 4–6).

Indeed, the construction of categories and observations of their members by outsiders may prompt vociferous challenges, as explained by Merton (1996: 330–331):

[T]he [Insider/Outsider] doctrine holds that the Outsider has a structurally imposed incapacity to comprehend alien groups, statuses, cultures, and societies. Unlike the Insider, the Outsider has neither been socialized in the group nor has engaged in the run of experience that makes up its life, and therefore cannot have the direct, intuitive sensitivity that alone makes empathic understanding possible. Only through continued socialization in the life of a group can one become fully aware of its symbolisms and socially shared realities; only so one can understand the fine-grained meanings of behavior, feelings, and values; only so one can decipher the unwritten grammar of conduct and the nuances of cultural idiom.

Shifting perceptions of self-identity and self-worth may also result in inconsistent self-designation across time and circumstance (Siegel and Passel, 1979; Snipp, 1986).

These classification schema and the discrepancies that they create underscore the difficulty of applying the concept of race, however it is defined. They also lend credence to the observation that "race is a societally constructed taxonomy that reflects the intersection of particular historical conditions with economic, political, legal, social, and cultural factors, as well as racism" (Williams, LaVizzo-Mourey, and Warren, 1994: 28).

History is replete with examples of medical judgments, medical care, and medical research that have been premised on differentiation between groups of people based on race. The pro-slavery physician John H. van Evrie claimed in his work entitled, *Negroes and Negro "Slavery": The First and Inferior Race; The Latter Its Normal Condition*, that dark skin resulted in an inability to express the full range of emotions, while the overall structure of the black spine obviated the ability to assume a directly perpendicular posture (Tucker, 1994). Dr. Samuel Cartwright, charged with the responsibility by the Medical Association of Louisiana of investigating and reporting on "the diseases and physical peculiarities of the Negro race," recommended as a cure for drapetomania, "the disease of the mind that caused slaves to run away to freedom" (Tucker, 1994: 14), that blacks be treated like children as long as they remained submissive, but have "the devil [whipped] out of them" if they dared to "raise their heads to a level with their master" (Cartwright, 1851: 892).

The Tuskegee syphilis study, as it has come to be known, is perhaps one of the most infamous and extreme examples of the use of race as the basis for medical research. In 1929, the United States Public Health Service (USPHS) conducted a study to examine the prevalence of syphilis among blacks and possible mechanisms for treatment. The town of Tuskegee, located in Macon County, Alabama, was found to have the highest rate of syphilis among the six counties that had been included in the study (Gill, 1932; Jones, 1981). This study, funded by the Julius Rosenwald Fund, concluded that mass treatment of syphilis would be feasible. However, funding became inadequate for the continuation of the project and the implementation of the treatment due to the economic depression that commenced in 1929 and which devastated the Fund's resources (Thomas and Quinn, 1991).

The Tuskegee syphilis study was initiated in 1932 by the USPHS to follow the natural history of untreated, latent syphilis in black males. The impetus for the study derived, in part, from conflict between the prevailing scientific view in the United States of the progression of syphilis in blacks and the results of a Norwegian study. In the U.S., it was believed that syphilis affected the cardiovascular system in blacks and neurological functioning in whites. In contrast, the Norwegian investigation found from its retrospective study of untreated syphilis in white men that the cardiovascular effects of the infection were common and the neurological consequences were relatively rare (Clark and Danbolt, 1955). However, even at the time that the Tuskegee study was initiated, there existed general consensus within the scientific community that syphilis required treatment even in its latent stages, despite the toxic effects of treatment. One venereologist of the day had stated with regard to treatment:

Though it imposes a slight though measurable risk of its own, treatment markedly diminishes the risk from syphilis. In latent syphilis... the probability of progression, relapse, or death is reduced from a probable 25–30 percent without treatment to about 5 percent with it; and the gravity of relapse if it occurs, is markedly diminished (Moore, 1933: 237).

Researchers believed that other racial differences existed as well. Blacks were said to possess an excessive sexual desire, a lack of morality (Hazen, 1914; Quillian, 1906), and an attraction to white women as the result of "racial instincts that are about as amenable to ethical culture as is the inherent odor of the race . . ." (Howard, 1903: 424).

The original Tuskegee study was designed to include black men between the ages of 25 and 60 who were infected with syphilis. The study protocol required a physical examination, x-rays, and a spinal tap. The original design did not include treatment for those men enrolled in the study, despite the existence of consensus in the medical community regarding the necessity of treatment (Brandt, 1985). Those men who were recruited for the study were told that they were ill with "bad blood," a euphemism that referred to syphilis, and that they would be provided with appropriate treatment and care. The mercurial ointment and neoarsphenamine provided to them as treatment were ineffective and were intended to be such. The researchers portrayed the spinal tap, which was administered for research purposes only, as a form of "special treatment" in order to encourage the men's participation. The investigators added a control group of healthy, uninfected men to the study as controls in 1933, following USPHS approval to continue with the study (Brandt, 1985).

The researchers detailed the conditions that made the study possible: follow-up by a nurse who was known to the men and who had come from the community from which they were recruited; the provision of burial assistance, not otherwise affordable by those enrolled in the study, as an incentive to continue participation; transportation provided by the nurse; and government sponsorship of what the men believed was care (Rivers, Schuman, Simpson, and Olansky, 1953).

The Tuskegee study continued for 40 years, despite the advent of numerous events that one would have thought would bring about its termination. First, the USPHS had begun to administer penicillin to some syphilitic patients in various treatment clinics (Mahoney et al., 1944). By at least 1945, it was clear in the professional literature that syphilis infections would respond to penicillin, including those cases that had been resistant to treatment with bismuth subsalicylate and mapharsen, a then-standard treatment (Noojin, Callaway, and Flower, 1945). However, the men of Tuskegee were not provided with this treatment and, in some instances, were even actively prevented by the research team from obtaining it (Thomas and Quinn, 1991).

Second, a series of articles published in professional journals indicated that the infected men were suffering to a much greater degree than the controls, with increased morbidity and a reduction in life expectancy (Deibert and Bruyere, 1946; Heller and Bruyere, 1946; Pesare, Bauer, and Gleeson, 1950; Vonderlehr, Clark, Wenger, and Heller, 1936). However, those who defended the study asserted, as late as 1974, that an inadequate basis existed to justify treatment with penicillin or with other regimens during the course of the study and that it was the "*shibboleth* of informed consent . . . born in court decisions in California (1957) and Kansas (1960)" that had provoked the controversy that surrounded the study (Kampmeier, 1974: 1352).

Finally, in 1949 the Nuremberg trials resulted in the production of the Nuremberg Code, which enunciated already-existing basic ethical principles to guide scientific research and researchers. These standards should have caused the investigators involved with the Tuskegee study to question the propriety of continuing the study, if not its initiation. This did not come to pass.

It was not until 1972 that the then-existing Department of Health, Education, and Welfare, in response to media criticism of the experiment, convened an advisory panel to evaluate the wisdom of continuing with the study (Brandt, 1985). The report of the committee focused on the failure to provide the enrolled men with penicillin to treat their infection and with the failure to obtain informed consent for participation in an experiment. According to Brandt (1985), this emphasis obscured the historical facts regarding the availability of drug treatment prior to the advent of penicillin, ignored the fact that the men had been led to believe that they were receiving clinical care, and failed to acknowledge that the men had unwittingly and unknowingly been used in an experiment (Brandt, 1985).

The Tuskegee study has become, for many blacks, a "symbol of their mistreatment by the medical establishment, a metaphor for deceit, conspiracy, malpractice, and neglect, if not outright racial genocide" (Jones, 1992: 38). Indeed, the conduct of the Tuskegee study and the associated efforts to deny the enrolled men adequate care have fostered significant distrust of the medical establishment within African American communities (Jones, 1992; Klonoff and Landrine, 1989; Thomas and Quinn, 1991).

Attempts to distinguish classes of persons on the basis of race were not, however, limited to blacks. Many of these supposed distinctions were utilized as the basis for the formulation of policies that often further marginalized and stigmatized the groups involved. As an example, the reported association between the Chinese and leprosy fueled a belief in the superiority of the "Anglo-Saxon race" and ultimately led to the formulation and implementation of restrictions on Chinese immigration to the United States and the exclusion of individuals with leprosy (Gussow, 1989). One writer observed,

At the present day Louisiana is threatened with an influx of Chinese and Malays, with filth, rice [sic] and leprous diseases. An inferior and barbarous race transferred from the burning heats of Africa has already been the occasion of the shedding of the blood of more than one million of the white inhabitants of the United States, and in the shock of arms and in the subsequent confusion and chaos attending the settlement of the question of African slavery, the liberties of the country have been well nigh destroyed, and it is but just that patriots should contemplate with dread the overflow of their country by the unprincipled, vicious and leprous bodies of Asia. The contact of a superior race with an inferior race must lead eventually to two results: The annihilation of one or the other, or the amalgamation of the two. The mixture of the blood of a noble race with that of one of the inferior mental and moral constitution may depress the former to the level of the latter, but can never endow the brain and heart of the African and Asiatic with the intelligence, independence, love of liberty, invention and moral worth of the Anglo-Saxon race (Jones, 1887: 1246–1247).

The formulation of policy on the basis of racial classification has not been confined to the United States. Indeed, "racial" categories provided the foundation for much of Hitler's agenda. The observations of Konrad Lorenz, who was awarded the Nobel Prize for his work in ethology, laid the groundwork for what was to be the Final Solution to rid Germany of its Jews, who were deemed to be of a "parasitic race" that represented a "biological danger" to the German people (Tucker, 1994: 127):

On the one hand, bodies with a cancerous tumor, and, on the other hand, a people with unfit individuals among them. Just as in cancer . . . the best treatment is the earliest possible recognition and eradication of the growth as quickly as possible, the racial-hygienic defense against genetically afflicted elements must be restricted to measures equally drastic . . . . [I]n the same way as the cells of a malignant tumor spread throughout the larger organism, [these elements would] pervade and destroy the healthy social body (Lorenz, 1940:68, 69).

Ethnicity, Ethnic Identity, and Ethnic Identification

Defining the Concepts

Ethnicity has been variously defined as the "self-identification and the identification by others of membership in a distinct socio-cultural group based on specific national and/or biological characteristics" (Melville, 1988: 76) and "the degree of conformity by members of the collectivity to . . . shared norms in the course of social interaction" (Cohen, 1974, in Sollors, 1996: 370). Ethnicity has also been described as a function of both cultural history and psychological identity (Melville, 1988), which "does not occur where the sociocultural environment is homogenous" (Melville, 1988: 76). Cooper (1994) distinguished between race and ethnicity by defining race as a biologic, rather than social, construct related to a single breeding population, with the resulting racial classifications premised on superficial phenotypic traits. In contrast, ethnicity was said to constitute "the relevant form of raciation among a species where cultural differentiation predominates," and is produced through social evolution as the product of genes, culture, and social class.

Weber defined *ethnic groups* as "human groups (other than kinship groups) which cherish a belief in their common origins of such kind that it provides a basis for the creation of a community" (Runciman, 1964: 364). Cohen's definition of ethnic group offers somewhat more specificity:

[A]n ethnic group can be operationally defined as a collectivity of people who (a) share some patterns of normative behaviour and (b) form a part of a larger population, interacting with people from other collectivities within the framework of a social system . . . By patterns of normative behaviour I am referring here to the symbolic formations and activities found in such contexts as kinship and marriage, friendship, rituals, and other types of ceremonial (Cohen, 1974, in Sollors, 1996: 370–371).

The *Harvard Encyclopedia of American Ethnic Groups* identified more than 100 distinct groups based on characteristics such as geographic origin, language, race, religion, neighborhood, traditions and values, food preferences, settlement patterns, an internal sense of distinctiveness, and an external perception of distinctiveness, among others (Thernstrom, 1980). As seen from these definitions, ethnicity may consist of both objective components, such as shared language and geographic origin, and subjective components, such as food preferences and an internal sense of distinctiveness.

The concept of "ethnic group" is inextricably linked to our understanding of culture. Like the delineation of ethnic boundaries, which comes about through the interplay of members and nonmembers of a specific group, the culture of an ethnic group is constructed through the interplay between group members and the larger society (Pereira de Queiroz, 1986). Nagel's (1994: 162) explanation is instructive:

[W]e have a useful device for examining the construction of ethnic culture: the shopping cart. We can think of ethnic boundary construction as determining the shape of the shopping cart (size, number of wheels, composition, etc.); ethnic culture, then, is composed of the things we put into the cart—art, music, dress, religion, norms, beliefs, symbols, myths, customs. It is important that we discard the notion that culture is simply an historical legacy; culture is not a shopping cart that came to us already loaded with a set of historical cultural goods. Rather we construct culture by picking and choosing items from the shelves of the past and the present... In other words, cultures change; they are borrowed, blended, rediscovered, and reinterpreted.... Culture is constructed in much the same way as ethnic boundaries are built, by the actions of individuals and groups and their interactions with the larger society. Ethnic boundaries function to determine identity options, membership composition and size, and form of ethnic organization. Boundaries answer the question: Who are we? Culture provides the content and meaning of ethnicity; it animates and authenticates ethnic boundaries by providing a history, ideology, symbolic universe, and system of meaning. Culture answers the question: What are we?

Too often, culture is erroneously assumed to be synonymous with ethnicity and then, in a leap of faith, is identified as the cause of a particular health condition. Karlsen (2004: 108–109) has explained how this occurs:

Studies which attempt to explore the relationship between ethnicity and health traditionally use measures of ethnicity based on country of origin and skin colour. This situation is partly a consequence of an assumption dominant in epidemiological research that the ethnic differentials found among various social and economic characteristics are a consequence of innate characteristics related to 'ethnic' or 'racial' difference: that ethnic differences are to some extent natural... [E]pidemiological research in this area has typically adopted an 'untheorised' approach, where culture is mapped onto reified ethnic categories and essentialized... While being presented as an empirically driven approach, the associated methodology and interpretation presume that 'ethnic/race' variables represent true and fixed genetic or cultural differences between groups, which lead to differences in health across groups. These genetic or cultural differences are, however, often assumed—after 'controlling for the existence of other influences—rather than directly measured... And the interpretations which follow are often made on the basis of ethnic stereotypes. As a consequence, culture itself becomes the *cause* of health differentials.... (Italics in original.)

Various concepts derive from that of ethnicity. Devereux (1975) provided a cogent definition of *ethnic identity*: "(1) A is an X...(2) A is not a non-X..." (Devereux, in Sollors, 1996: 397). Yinger (1994: 3–4) identified three elements critical to ethnic identity:

(1) The group is perceived by others in the society to be different in some combination of the following traits: language, religion, race, and ancestral homeland with its related culture; (2) the members also perceive themselves as different; and (3) they participate in shared activities built around their (real or mythical) common origin and culture.

Ethnic identity may refer to membership in a tribe, region, race, or nation (Yinger, 1994).

Ethnic identity, then, arises from the interplay between what the individual believes his or her identity to be and what others believe his or her ethnicity to be (Barth, 1969). That identity may be multi-layered and may encompass subtribal, tribal, regional, or supra-tribal identities, as is the case with Native Americans (Cornell, 1988), or ethnic, pan-ethnic, and nationality-based identities, as is the case among Latino (Gimenez, Lopez, and Munoz, Jr., 1992; Padilla, 1985, 1986), Asian American (Espiritu, 1992), and African American groups (Waters, 1990).

Nahirny and Fishman (1965, in Sollors, 1996: 269) distinguished between *ethnic identification*, "a person's use of racial, national or religious terms to identify himself, and thereby, to relate himself to others," and *ethnic orientation*, meaning "those features of a person's feeling and action towards others which are a function of the ethnic category by which he identifies himself."

The concept of race has often been confused or intertwined with that of ethnicity (cf. Yinger, 1994). Consider the following definitions of *race*.

[A race] is a vast family of human beings, generally of common blood and language, always of common history, traditions, and impulses, who are both voluntarily and involuntarily striving together for the accomplishment of certain more or less vividly conceived ideals of life (DuBois, 1897: 7).

1. an ethnic stock, or division of mankind; in a narrower sense, a national or tribal stock; in a still narrower sense, a genealogic line of descent; a class of persons of common lineage. In genetics, races are considered as populations having different distributions of gene frequencies. 2. a class or breed of animals; a groups of individuals having certain characteristics in common, owing to a common inheritance; a subspecies (Taylor, 1988).

Van den Burghe (1967:9) noted the confusion in distinguishing between the concepts of race and ethnicity as they are used:

In practice, the distinction between a racial and ethnic group is sometimes blurred by several facts. Cultural traits are often regarded as genetic and inherited (e.g., body odor, which is a function of diet, cosmetics, and other cultural items); physical appearance can be culturally changed (by scarification, surgery, and cosmetics); and the sensory perception of physical differences is affected by cultural perceptions of race (e.g., a rich Negro may be seen as lighter than an equally dark poor Negro, as suggested by the Brazilian proverb: "Money bleaches.")

Several recent research studies serve to highlight the confusion that often attends efforts to classify individuals by race and/or ethnicity A study of hospitalizations in Rhode Island during the period stemming from 1990 through 2003 found that, during this time, hospitals utilized three different formats for race and ethnicity data and some of the formats required that ethnicity and race be collapsed into single categories (Buechner, 2004). Through September 1998, individuals were classified as white, black, Asian or Pacific Islander, American Indian or Alaskan Native, other, or not reported. From October 1998 through March 2003, the following categories were utilized: white Hispanic, white not Hispanic, black Hispanic, black not Hispanic, Asian or Pacific Islander, American Indian or Alaskan Native, other, and not reported. Beginning in April 2003, a distinction was made between race and ethnicity. Ethnicity was reported as Hispanic, not Hispanic, or not reported, while race was recorded as white, black, Asian, American Indian or Alaska Native, Native Hawaiian or other Pacific Islander, other, or not reported.

Yet another study focusing on the use of race- and ethnic group-related terms in the Medical Subject Headings (MeSH) that are used to index articles in the MEDLINE database found that the definitions are outdated and inconsistent (Sankar, 2003). MeSH refers to "racial stocks," defined as "major living subspecies of man differentiated by genetic and physical characteristics" (Sankar, 2003: 119). Four races are listed: Caucasoid, Mongoloid, Negroid, and Australoid. "Ethnic groups" are defined as "a group of people with a common cultural heritage that sets them apart from others in a variety of social relationships" (Sankar, 2003: 119). The 13 enumerated ethnic groups are defined based on their geographic location, racial classification, ancestry, and/or history. Racial stocks are said to refer to the physical and genetic characteristics of a population, whereas "ethnic group" is said to encompass psychological, social, cultural, ethnological, or sociological features of a population. It has been found that as many as 30% of the articles that conform with the stated criteria for "racial stock" are actually indexed by ethnic group (Sankar, 2003).

The British census seems to similarly collapses race and ethnicity in many of its categories and, in addition, utilizes information pertaining to nationality in classifying individuals (Riddell-Heaney, 2001). These categories are as follows:

- White: British, Irish, or any other white background
- Mixed: White and black Caribbean, white and black African, white and Asian, any other mixed background
- Asian: Asian, Asian British, any other Asian background
- Black: Black, black British, any other black background
- Chinese: As evidenced by skin color and other aspects of physical appearance
- Nationality: Derived from country of birth or citizenship
- Any other ethnic groups

Under this classification, one must wonder how a person with white skin who was born in a Scandinavian country and holds citizenship in a Southeast Asian country would be classified. The possibilities include Asian, white, mixed (based on nationality), Norwegian (country of birth), and Thai (country of citizenship).

Both ethnic and racial identity depend upon one's subjective personal knowledge about one's group and pride in membership (Aboud and Doyle, 1993). Three psychological components of ethnic identity have been suggested: self-identification, a recognition of oneself as different from other ethnic groups, and a perception that ethnicity is constant (Aboud, 1988). Behaviors, such as traditions, customs, and language, may also be critical to ethnic identity (Knight, Tein, Shell, and Roosa, 1993). Ethnic identity persists through the process of socialization into the specific culture (Oetting, Swaim, and Chiarella, 1998), a process known as *enculturation* (Knight, Tein, Shell, and Roosa, 1993). This process occurs with respect to both the dominant culture and the subgroup culture.

Specific models have been developed to better understand and explain ethnic or racial identity within specific groups. As an example, Cross and colleagues have developed a model to explain the formulation of black identity. They have hypothesized that individuals progress through four stages: preencounter, encounter, immersion-emersion, and internalization (Cross, Parham, and Helms, 1985, 1991; Parham and Williams, 1993). During the preencounter stage, individuals are either clearly pro-white or pro-black. The encounter stage involves a reevaluation of these attitudes and an evolution towards the third stage of immersion-emersion, during which individuals are more pro-black and anti-white. Ultimately, the individual develops a more pluralistic perspective during the internalization phase. Individuals may begin at any point on this continuum and may recycle through the various stages.

The Cross model reflects the similarities across numerous models relating to the development of black identity. Common characteristics include (1) beliefs about being black (views towards other African Americans, cultural pride, affinity for things perceived as black, the adoption of Afrocentric values); (2) attitudes towards whites (preferences towards having whites as friends, views of intermarriage and living in mixed neighborhoods); and (3) recognition and perception of racism at the level of individuals, institutions, and society (Resnicow, Soler, Braithwaite, Selassie, and Smith, 1999).

Instruments that require respondents to select from among preconstructed categories of ethnicity offer the advantage of confining responses to a predetermined number of options ("forced-choice situations"), thereby limiting the number of diverse classifications, which may facilitate statistical analysis. However, this approach may engender a variety of difficulties (Evinger, 1995; Stanfield, 1993). First, because the respondents did not choose the categories themselves to describe who they are, some respondents may decide that they do not fit into any of the preformulated groups. As an example, 57% of the respondents to a survey conducted in the San Luis Valley area of Colorado self-identified as "Other," rather than "Hispanic," because they considered themselves "Spanish," rather than "Hispanic," due to their ability to trace their ancestry to the 17th century Spanish colonists who had settled in that area (Pappas, 1993). (Instruments related to cultural and racial identity and identification are discussed in additional depth in chapter 6.)

Second, the preformulated categories may carry political connotations that influence individuals' identification with them. Still other categories may be confusing or ambiguous. Estrada's research relating to then-existing census categories for individuals of Mexican-origin revealed that

1. Native-born Mexican-origin persons still react negatively to the "hyphenated American category" . . . feeling that it represents marginalization.
2. Older Mexican-origin persons still react strongly to the term "Chicano," and do not like to be associated with that term . . . based on the activist groups associated with the term and what some regard as a "street language" term.
3. "Mexican" and "Mexican American" are often used by Mexican-origin persons to distinguish between Mexico-born and U.S.-born persons, although that was not the intention of them. Thus, Mexican-born parents self-identify as Mexican, but they list their children as Mexican American if they were born in the U.S.
4. Recent analysis of a . . . expanded race items . . . showed that a number of Hispanics identified themselves and their children as Asian and Pacific Islanders, having mistakenly marked the item "Laotian" in the race item, obviously confusing it for "Latino" (Estrada, 1993: 175–176).

The perceived social consequences associated with specific ethnicities may also be critical to how one self-identifies. Melville (1988: 75) explained:

What is so embarrassing about being Mexican? Why would anyone want to say they were Colombian or Spanish rather than Mexican? . . . The presumption is that if you are Colombian, you came to the U. S. by airplane, you could pay your own way, were somewhat sophisticated, probably of middle- or upper-class. If you are Mexican, on the other hand, the presumption is that you or your ancestors swam across the Rio Grande or climbed over the fence in California, were penniless, and have been working as unskilled or farm laborers ever since. By saying that one is Colombian, rather than Mexican, one establishes social class rather than ethnic identity.

Because the social context of one's identity changes, one's self-categorization may also change over time (cf. Velez-Ibáñez, 1996). Limerick (1995: 27) postulated that

[b]y defining and claiming an ethnic identity individuals try to place themselves in large currents of life, try to find a sense of destiny and purpose, and try to get out, at least momentarily, from under the burden of being isolated individuals responsible for their own self-definition and direction at every moment.

As an example of how the social context of ethnic identification may change over time, consider Melville's explanation, which she offered in 1988. In view of the U.S. "War on Drugs" and the continuous press coverage of Colombian drug lords and the drug-related violence in Colombia (BBC, 2005; Kirk, 2003), it would not be surprising if similarly disparaging stereotypes now existed with respect to individuals of Colombian ethnicity, that is, that if they are middle- or upper-class, it must be a result of their ties to drug traffickers and participation in drug trafficking.

The extent to which individuals acknowledge all or parts of their heritage is also related to how they feel about that heritage. Nahirny and Fishman (1965, in Sollors, 1996: 273) explained:

The more intensely [the sons of immigrants] despised their ethnic heritage the more conscious they were of their ethnic identity. The more ashamed they were of their past, and even of their parents, the more they were aware of their ethnic background. For it should be kept in mind that by suppressing ethnicity the sons also rebelled against parts of themselves.

Immigration Status

Like ethnicity, "foreignnesss" has often been equated with race. Consider the following examples.

Mussolini's Italy was characterized by significant diversity. Attempts to solidify and maintain power were often masked by nationalistic appeals to ethnic purity. A 1938 manifesto distributed throughout Italy proclaimed:

The root of differences among peoples and nations is to be found in differences of race. If Italians differ from Frenchmen, Germans, Turks, Greeks, etc., this is not just because they possess a different language and different history, but because their racial development is different.... A pure 'Italian race' is already in existence. This pronouncement [rests] on the very pure blood tie that unites present-day Italians.... This ancient purity of blood is the Italian nation's greatest title of nobility (Quoted in Delzell, 1970: 193–194).

Rudolph Pintner, a professor at Columbia Teachers College, concluded in a study in 1923 that "the races from the south and east of Europe seem inferior in intelligence to those from the north and west." He explained the social significance of his findings by stating:

Mental ability is inherited. The population of the United States is largely recruited by immigration. The country cannot afford to admit year after year large numbers of mentally inferior people, who will continue to multiply and lower the level of intelligence of the whole nation. Our tests, although inconclusive, would seem to indicate that the level of certain racial groups coming to this country is below that of the nation at large. Increased vigilance is, therefore, required (Pintner, 1923: 362).

This putative association between intelligence and immigration, which served as a euphemism for race, was further reinforced by the work of Carl C. Brigham, a professor of psychology at Princeton University and the author of *A Study of American Intelligence*. Brigham analyzed the results of intelligence tests administered to foreign-born persons in the United States. He found that the average test score increased as the number of years of residence in the U.S. increased. He rejected the notion that these differences might be attributable to linguistic, educational, or cultural factors and concluded, instead, that the country had experienced "a gradual deterioration in the class of immigrants" to its shores during the previous two decades. Brigham trichotomized the European immigrants into three racial groups: the Nordics, who were said to be fair-haired and blue-eyed; the Mediterraneans, who were described as short and dark-eyed; and the Alpines, stocky and brown-eyed. He then provided racial estimates for the "present blood constitution" of the immigrants from each of the European countries from which they had migrated. As an example, Swedes were judged to be 100% Nordic, while

Asian Turks were determined to be 90% Mediterranean and European Turks were 40% Mediterranean and 60% Alpine (Brigham, 1923).

Robert Yerkes, a staunch advocate of eugenics and the architect of the intelligence test utilized by the army during World War I, explained:

If we may safely judge by the army measurements of intelligence, races are quite as significantly different as individuals ... [and] almost as great as the intellectual difference between negro and white in the army are the differences between white racial groups ....

For the past ten years or so the intellectual status of immigrants has been disquietingly low. Perhaps this is because of the dominance of the Mediterranean races, as contrasted with the Nordic and Alpine (Quoted in Carlson and Colburn, 1972: 333–334).

More recently, the politics of HIV/AIDS illustrates the interplay between conceptualizations of race, ethnicity, and immigration, and the impact of such assumptions on disease definition and prevention. The disease condition now known as AIDS, for acquired immunodeficiency syndrome, was first labeled as such in 1982. The causative agent of the disease, the human immunodeficiency virus (HIV), is transmitted through the exchange of various body fluids, such as blood, semen, and vaginal secretions. Although the virus can be isolated in tears, sweat, and saliva, it has not been shown to be transmitted via these fluids. Transmission occurs through transfusion with contaminated blood or blood products; through transplantation with an infected organ; through unprotected sexual intercourse, including oral intercourse; through the use of contaminated injection equipment, including needles, syringes, cookers, and cotton; and through vertical transmission from mother to child. Transmission and progression of the disease may be accelerated by various factors including a co-occurring sexually transmitted infection (Abrams, 1997; Volberding, 1997).

Initially, research relating to HIV/AIDS focused on the identification of routes of transmission and risk factors for the disease. By 1982, within a year of identifying the first cases of what would come to be called AIDS, the Centers for Disease Control and Prevention (CDC) had labeled Haitians a "risk group." This emphasis on group membership as a risk factor, rather than relevant activities or behaviors, ultimately resulted in the medical and social construction of "risk groups," whose members were presumed to be at higher risk of contracting and transmitting the infection by virtue of their membership in the specified group, regardless of their individual behaviors (Schiller, Crystal, and Lewellen, 1994). These four groups— Haitians, homosexuals, heroin addicts, and hemophiliacs—came to be known as "the 4-H club."

Like the concepts of race and ethnicity, however, who is to be considered an immigrant and what constitutes immigration is the focus of considerable debate. Essentially, three paradigms exist for the definition of immigrant and the determination of immigrant status: social science, immigration law, and public benefit entitlement.

In the context of social science, migration has been defined as

the physical transition of an individual or a group from one society to another. This transition usually involves abandoning one social setting and entering a different one (Eisenstadt, 1955: 1) a relatively permanent moving away of . . . migrants, from one geographical location to another, preceded by decision-making on the part of the migrants on the basis of a hierarchically ordered set of values or valued ends and resulting in changes in the interactional set of migrants (Mangalam, 1968: 8)

a permanent or semipermanent change of residence (Lee, 1966:49)

These definitions assume that an individual classifiable as an immigrant retains that characterization or label regardless of the duration of his or her residence in the new geographical location and that there are commonalities across all migrating groups and individuals that justify their classification together as immigrants, regardless of the context or legality of their migration. Indeed, the appropriateness of characterizing specific groups as immigrants may depend on the nature of the research to be undertaken. For instance, Spanish-speaking Puerto Ricans born on the island of Puerto Rico could be considered immigrants if one were examining language barriers to care among residents of New York City. However, a study seeking to examine differences between immigrants and non-immigrants in the utilization of Medicaid-funded health services would presumably consider Puerto Ricans within the category of not-immigrants, as their eligibility for such services is similar to that of mainland U.S.-born individuals.

Unlike the social science definition, the immigration law paradigm distinguishes between groups of individuals based upon their place of birth and the basis for their presence in the United States. All individuals who are not citizens are considered to be aliens; aliens can be present in the United States temporarily or permanently, legally or illegally, with or without documentation of their status. These characteristics are not synonymous. For instance, an individual may be a citizen, legally present in the United States but without documentation; U.S. citizens are not required by law to maintain proof of their citizenship. An individual may be undocumented, having entered the country illegally, but still be a citizen, having derived U.S. citizenship from his or her parents. An individual who has applied for asylum in the United States due to fear of persecution should he return to his own country is an immigrant within the social science paradigm, but within the immigration law paradigm, is neither a nonimmigrant (intending to remain temporarily) nor an immigrant (lacking legal status). Public benefit law adds further complexity by delineating both undocumented individuals and specified groups of legally immigrated individuals as ineligible for specified public benefits and creating a category of "qualified aliens," consisting of those noncitizens who are eligible for publicly-funded benefits (Personal Responsibility and Work Opportunity Reconciliation Act of 1996).

Acculturation, Cultural Identity, and Cultural Identification

The concept of acculturation has been used to distinguish within and across different ethnic and racial groups on the basis of their affinity to one or more cultures. Such distinctions may be important in the health context in relationship to groups' and subgroups' ability to access health care and efforts to prevent or ameliorate specific diseases and their symptoms within groups. For instance, acculturation level has been found to be associated with the use of tobacco, alcohol and other drugs (Otero-Sabogal, Sabogal, and Perez-Stable, 1995) and with the use of preventive health services (Harmon, Castro, and Coe, 1996).

Acculturation has been conceived of as

[comprehending] those phenomena which result when groups of individuals having different cultures come into continuous first-hand contact, with subsequent changes in the original culture patterns of either or both groups.... Under this definition acculturation is to be distinguished from culture change, of which it is but one aspect, and assimilation, which is at times a phase of acculturation. It is also to be differentiated from diffusion, which while occurring in all instances of acculturation, is only a phenomena which frequently takes place without the occurrence of the types of contact between people specified in the definition above, but also constitutes only one aspect of the process of acculturation (Redfield, Linton, and Herskovits, 1936).

culture change that is initiated by the conjunction of two or more autonomous cultural systems. Acculturative change may be the consequence of direct cultural transmission; it may be derived from noncultural causes, such as ecological or demographic modifications, induced by an impinging culture; it may be delayed, as with internal adjustments following upon the acceptance of alien traits or patterns; or it may be a reactive adaptation of traditional modes of life. Its dynamics can be seen as the selective adaptation of value systems, the processes of integration and differentiation, the generation of developmental sequences, and the operation of role determinants and personality factors (Social Science Research Council, 1954: 974).

At one time, acculturation was conceived of as occurring along a continuum, from unacculturated (to the dominant culture) at one extreme to completely acculturated (to the dominant culture) at the other (Keefe and Padilla, 1987). At the center of these two extremes were individuals who were considered bicultural, or equally acculturated to both the dominant culture and their "ethnic" subgroup culture. (This presumes, of course, that only those who are not members of the dominant culture, whatever it may be, are "ethnic" and ignores the reality that everyone is of some ethnicity.) This model presumes that acculturation is a unidirectional process in which groups lose their affinity and connection to their culture of origin and gradually assume the traits of the dominant culture.

Other models of acculturation recognize to a greater extent and in differing degrees the complexity of the process. The two-culture model assumes that individuals can be highly acculturated or relatively unacculturated simultaneously in both their culture of origin and their newly acquired culture (Keefe and Padilla, 1987; McFee, 1968). The multidimensional model of acculturation recognizes that groups may simultaneously retain elements of their culture of origin, while adopting the traits of their new milieu. Accordingly, the level of acculturation can be said to be specific to identified traits (Keefe and Padilla, 1987).

The process of acculturation has been theorized to consist of various forms (Broom, Sigel, Vogt, Watson, and Barnett, 1954; Berry, 1993). *Diffusion* refers to the selective adaptation of specific cultural elements, such as traits or ideas, between two systems. *Cultural creativity*, also known as syncretism, is the process by which new cultural constructions occur, such as the construction of an analogy with Draino, a modern concept, to explain the action of the traditional remedy *pamita* (tansy mustard) in curing *empacho*, "the clogging of the intestines" (Clark and Hofsess, 1998: 44). *Cultural disintegration* requires that subgroup members choose between irreconcilable differences between views or behaviors of the dominant culture and those of their culture of origin. The term *reactive adaptation* is used to describe the process by which groups reaffirm and reinforce their traditional values as a reaction to the dominant culture.

The process of acculturation has been depicted as consisting of three distinct phases: contact, conflict, and adaptation (Berry, 1980). The contact can occur through a variety of means, including trade, communications, and invasion. Conflict will occur as the less dominant group resists the loss of valued features of its culture. Adaptation provides a means by which the conflict may be reduced or stabilized and can take a number of forms, including adjustment, reaction, and withdrawal.

As indicated, acculturation is distinguishable from *assimilation*, which refers to individuals' complete absorption and integration into one culture from another. This allows full participation in the economic, social, and political life of the culture in which they have assimilated (Gordon, 1964; Keefe and Padilla, 1987), but also results in the relinquishing of cultural identity (Berry, 1980; Rose, 1956). Seven facets of assimilation have been identified:

1. cultural/behavioral assimilation, also known as acculturation, which represents a change in cultural patterns;
2. structural assimilation, or the large-scale entrance of the immigrants into the institutions of the receiving society;
3. marital assimilation, or amalgamation, meaning large-scale intermarriage between individuals in the receiving society and those of the migrant society;
4. identificational assimilation, referring to the development of a sense of peoplehood that rests on identification with the receiving society;
5. attitude receptional assimilation, or the absence of prejudice in the receiving society;
6. behavior receptional assimilation, or the absence of discrimination in the receiving society; and
7. civic assimilation, meaning the absence of value and power conflict (Gordon, 1964).

Each aspect of assimilation is believed to represent a spectrum or continuum.

Although not typically considered in conjunction with efforts to assess acculturation levels, these concepts of assimilation may be important in the context of assessing health, health care, and access issues. For instance, the concept of stigma in the context of immigrants' access to health care or barriers to access may be closely related to attitude receptional assimilation and behavior receptional assimilation in that one could hypothesize that an increase in these facets of assimilation would correspond to reduced levels of stigma and increased access to care.

Existing measures of acculturation differ with respect to the domains considered to reflect the process of acculturation. Those that have been utilized include language use (Deyo, Diehl, Hazuda, and Stern), cultural awareness and ethnic identification (Padilla, 1980), media preferences (Marín, Sabogal, Marín, Otero-Sabogal, and Peréz-Stable, 1987), social activities (Burnam, Hough, Karno, Telles, and Escobar, 1987), ethnic pride and affiliation, and/or ethnic identity (Keefe and Padilla, 1987). Chapter 6 provides a brief overview of some of these measures.

Some scholars have distinguished between cultural identity and *cultural identification*, explaining that a

cultural identity is a person's affiliation with a specific group. It is usually a qualitative classification of membership, and although it is usually a self-perception, in some cases it can be assigned by others...Membership in an ethnic group is one example of cultural identity....

In contrast with identity, cultural identification is a personal trait. It is the extent to which individuals view themselves as involved with an identifiable group along with their investment in or stake in that particular culture...Whereas cultural identity can be qualitative, cultural identification is quantitative; it assesses the strengths of a person's links to a particular culture (Oetting, Swaim, and Chiarella, 1998: 132).

Models of Cultural Identification

A variety of models have been developed in an attempt to explain how people adapt and change over time. Early models viewed the process of cultural identification as unidirectional, with movement from the culture of origin towards adaptation to the majority or dominant culture (Oetting, Swaim, and Chiarella, 1998). This model conceived of the majority culture as superior to the culture of origin, and a failure to move towards identification with the majority culture as a weakness. Not surprisingly, this model mirrors the unidimensional model of acculturation.

Transitional models posit that individuals may encounter problems as they move from one culture towards the majority culture; they are unable to utilize the strengths of their culture of origin, but are as yet unable to access the benefits and strengths of the dominant culture. The alienation model is somewhat similar, but does not rest on the assumption that individuals will necessarily experience difficulties in their transition from the culture of origin to the dominant culture (Graves, 1967).

Multidimensional models of cultural identification posit, in contrast, that movement occurs in a number of domains, such as language and loyalty (Olmedo, Martinez, and Martinez, 1978; Olmedo and Padilla, 1978). Change may occur in one or more of the domains and may occur at differing rates but, ultimately, individuals are said to exist somewhere between the two cultures. The bicultural model departs from this assumption, positing that individuals can be bicultural and that a bicultural individual has "extensive socialization and life experiences in two or more cultures and participates actively in these cultures. In addition, the behavior is flexible in the sense that he or she uses different problem solving, coping, human relational, communication, and incentive motivational styles" (Ramirez, 1984: 82).

The orthogonal model of cultural identification (Oetting, 1993; Oetting and Beauvais, 1990) is a cognate of Berry's model of acculturation. The orthogonal model posits independence in the extent of cultural identification with the cultures involved (Oetting, Swaim, and Chiarella, 1998). Accordingly, individuals may indicate a low level of identification with any culture, the same levels of identification with the cultures involved, or differing levels of identification across the relevant cultures.

Summary

The concepts of race, ethnicity, citizenship, alienage, and acculturation are associated and, at times, have been used interchangeably despite significant differences in their meaning. The referent groups encompassed by a specific category label have often varied across time, place, and culture. This inconsistent application of terms renders interpretation of studies difficult and may require the disentangling of meanings in order to compare findings across studies. This lack of clarity in the use of these terms has permeated both scientific research and policymaking. Although distinctions between groups on the basis of their characteristics may be necessary in order to develop targeted health intervention programs, these distinctions too often are without logical basis and may inadvertently provide the foundation for discriminatory action.

References

Aboud, F. (1988). *Children and Prejudice*. New York: Blackwell.

Aboud, F., Doyle, A.B. (1993). The early development of ethnic identity and attitudes. In M. Bernal, G.P. Knight (Eds.), *Ethnic Identity: Formation and Transmission among Hispanics and Other Minorities* (pp. 47–59). Albany, New York: State University of New York Press.

Barth, F. (1969). *Ethnic Group and Boundaries*. Boston: Little, Brown.

BBC. (2005). Q & A: Colombia's civil conflict. BBC News, UK edition, May 24. Available at http://news.bbc.co.uk/1/hi/world/americas/1738963.stm. Last accessed September 13, 2005.

Becker, E.L., Landav, S.I. (1992). *Health Issues in the Black Community*. San Francisco: Jossey-Bass Publishers.

Berry, J. (1993). Ethnic identity in plural societies. In M. Bernal, G. Knight (Eds.), *Ethnic Identity: Formation and Transmission among Hispanics and Other Minorities* (pp. 271–296). Albany, New York: State University of New York Press.

Berry, J.W. (1980). Acculturation as varieties of adaptation. In A. Padilla (Ed.), *Acculturation Theory, Models, and Some New Findings* (pp. 9–25). Boulder, Colorado: Westview Press.

Boas, F. (1940). *Race, Language, and Culture*. New York: Free Press.

Brandt, A.M. (1985). Racism and research: The case of the Tuskegee syphilis study. In J.W. Leavitt, R.L. Numbers (Eds.), *Sickness and Health in America: Readings in the*

History of Medicine and Public Health (pp. 331–343). Madison, Wisconsin: University of Wisconsin Press.

Brigham, C.C. (1923). *A Study of American Intelligence*. Princeton, New Jersey: Princeton University Press.

Broom, L., Sigel, B.J., Vogt, E.Z., Watson, J.B., Barnett, B.H. (1954). Acculturation: An exploratory formulation. *American Anthropologist* 56: 973–1000.

Buechner, J.S. (2004). Hospitalizations by race and ethnicity, Rhode Island, 1990–2003. *Medicine and Health/Rhode Island* 87(7): 220–221.

Buescher, P.A., Gizlice, Z., Jones-Vessey, K.A. (2005). Discrepancies between published data on racial classification and self-reported race: Evidence from the 2002 North Carolina live birth records. *Public Health Reports* 120: 393–398.

Burnam, A.M., Hough, R.L., Karno, M., Telles, C.A., Escobar, J.I. (1987). Measurement of acculturation in a community population of Mexican Americans. *Journal of Behavioral Sciences* 9(2): 105–130.

Carlson, L.H., Colburn, G.A. (1972). *In Their Place: White America Defines Her Minorities, 1850–1950*. New York: Wiley.

Cartwright, S.A. (1851). Report on the diseases and physical peculiarities of the Negro race. *New Orleans Medical and Surgical Journal* 7: 692–693.

Clark, E.G., Danbolt, N. (1955). The Oslo study of the natural history of untreated syphilis. *Journal of Chronic Disease* 2: 311–344.

Clark, L., Hofsess, L. (1998). Acculturation. In S. Loue (Ed.), *Handbook of Immigrant Health* (pp. 37–59). New York: Plenum Press.

Cohen, A. (1974). The lesson of ethnicity (1974). In W. Sollors (Ed.), (1996). *Theories of Ethnicity: A Classical Reader* (pp. 370–384). New York: New York University Press.

Cross, W., Parham, T., Helms, J. (1985). Nigrescence revisited: Theory and research. In R. Jones (Ed.), *Advances in Black Psychology* (pp. 81–98). New York: Harper and Row.

Cross, W., Parham, T., Helms, J. (1991). The stages of Black identity development, Nigrescence models. In R. Jones (Ed.), *Black Psychology*, 3rd ed. (pp. 319–338). Berkeley, California: Cobb & Henry.

Davis, J.F. (1991). *Who Is Black? One Nation's Definition*. University Park, Pennsylvania: Pennsylvania State University Press.

Deibert, A.V., Bruyere, M.C. (1946). Untreated syphilis in the Negro male. III. Evidence of cardiovascular abnormalities and other forms of morbidity. *Journal of Venereal Disease Information* 27: 301–314.

Delzell, C. (1970). *Mediterranean Fascism*. New York: Harper & Row.

Devereux, G. (1975). Ethnic identity: Its logical foundations and its dysfunctions. In W. Sollors (Ed.), (1996). *Theories of Ethnicity: A Classical Reader* (pp. 385–414). New York: New York University Press.

Deyo, R.A. Diehl, A.K., Hazuda, H., Stern, M.P. (1985). A simple language-based acculturation scale for Mexican Americans: Validation and application to health care research. *American Journal of Public Health* 75(1): 51–55.

Dikötter, F. (2003). The discourse of race in modern China. In J. Stone, R. Dennis (Eds.), *Race and Ethnicity: Comparative and Theoretical Approaches* (pp. 125–135). Malden, Massachusetts: Blackwell Publishing.

Ehrlich, P.R., Feldman, S.S. (1977). *The Race Bomb*. New York: Quadrangle.

Eisenstadt, S.N. (1955). *The Absorption of Immigrants*. Glencoe, Illinois: Free Press.

Espiritu, Y. (1992). *Asian American Panethnicity: Bridging Institutions and Identities*. Philadelphia, Pennsylvania: Temple University Press.

Estrada, L.F. (1993). Family influences on demographic trends in Hispanic ethnic identi-fication and labeling. In M. Bernal, G.P. Knight (Eds.), *Ethnic Identity: Formation and Transmission among Hispanics and Other Minorities* (pp. 163–179). Albany, New York: State University of New York Press.

Gaines, A.D. (1994). Race and racism. In W. Reich (Ed.), *Encyclopedia of Bioethics*. New York: Macmillan.

Gill, D.G. (1932). Syphilis in the rural Negro: Results of a study in Alabama. *Southern Medical Journal* 25: 985–900.

Gimenez, M.E., Lopez, F.A., Munoz, C., Jr. (1992). *The Politics of Ethnic Construction: Hispanic, Chicano, Latino?* Beverly Hills, California: Sage Publications.

Gomez, S.L., Kelsey, J.L., Glaser, S.L., Lee, M.M., Sidney, S. (2005). Inconsistencies be-tween self-reported ethnicity and ethnicity recorded in a health maintenance organization. *Annals of Epidemiology* 15: 71–79.

Gordon, M.M. (1964). *Assimilation in American Life: The Role of Race, Religion, and National Origins*. New York: Oxford University Press.

Gould, S.J. (1981). *The Mismeasure of Man*. New York: W.W. Norton.

Graves, T.D. (1967). Psycholofical acculturation in a tri-ethnic community. *Southwestern Journal of Anthropology* 23: 337–350.

Gray v. Ohio, 4 Ohio 353 (1831).

Gussow, Z. (1989). *Leprosy, Racism, and Public Health: Social Policy in Chronic Disease Control*. Boulder, Colorado: Westview Press.

Hahn, R.A. (1992). The state of federal health statistics on racial and ethnic groups. *Journal of the American Medical Association* 267: 268–271.

Harmon, M.P., Castro, F.G., Coe, K. (1996). Acculturation and cervical cancer: Knowledge, beliefs, and behaviors of Hispanic women. *Women and Health* 24(3): 37–57.

Hazen, H.H. (1914). Syphilis in the American Negro. *Journal of the American Medical Association* 63: 463–466.

Heller, J.R., Bruyere, P.T. (1946). Untreated syphilis in the male Negro. II. Mortality during 12 years of observation. *Journal of Venereal Disease Information* 27: 34–38.

Howard, W.L. (1903). The Negro as a distinct ethnic factor in civilization. *Medicine (Detroit)* 9: 424.

Jaimes, M.A. (1994). American racism: Impact on American-Indian identity and survival. In S. Gregory, R. Sanjek (Eds.), *Race* (pp. 41–61). New Brunswick, New Jersey: Rutgers University Press.

Jaimes, M.A. (1990). Federal Indian Identification Policy, Ph.D. dissertation, Arizona State University.

Jay N. (1981). Gender and dichotomy. *Feminist Studies* 7: 38–56.

Jones, J. (1981). *Bad Blood: The Tuskegee Syphilis Experiment—A Tragedy of Race and Medicine*. New York: Free Press.

Jones, J. (1887). *Medical and Surgical Memoirs... 1855–1866* (Vol. 2). New Orleans. Quoted in Z. Gussow. (1989). *Leprosy, Racism, and Public Health: Social Policy in Chronic Disease Control*. Boulder, Colorado: Westview Press.

Kampmeier, R.H. (1974). Final report on the "Tuskegee syphilis study." *Southern Medical Journal* 67: 1349–1353.

Karlsen, S. (2004). 'Black like Beckham'? Moving beyond definitions of ethnicity based on skin colour and ancestry. *Ethnicity & Health* 9(2): 107–137.

Keefe, S., Padilla, A.M. (1987). *Chicano Ethnicity*. Albuquerque, New Mexico: University of New Mexico Press.

King, R.C., Stanfield, W.D. (1990). *A Dictionary of Genetics*. London: Oxford University Press.

Kirk, R. (2003). *More Terrible Than Death: Violence, Drugs, and America's War in Colombia*. New York: Public Affairs.

Klonoff, E.A., Landrine, H. (1999). Do blacks believe that HIV/AIDS is a government conspiracy against them? *Preventive Medicine* 28: 451–457.

Knight, G.P., Tein, J.Y., Shell, R., Roosa, M. (1993). Family socialization and Mexican American identity and behavior. In M. Bernal, G.P. Knight (Eds.), *Ethnic Identity: Formation and Transmission among Hispanics and Other Minorities* (pp. 105–129). Albany, New York: State University of New York Press.

Kressin, N.R., Chang, B-H., Hendricks, A., Kazis, L.E. (2003). Agreement between administrative data and patients' self-reports of race/ethnicity. *American Journal of Public Health* 93(10): 1734–1739.

Lancaster, R.N. (2003). Skin color, race, and racism in Nicaragua. In J. Stone, R. Dennis (Eds.), *Race and Ethnicity: Comparative and Theoretical Approaches* (pp. 98–113). Malden, Massachusetts: Blackwell Publishing.

Lauderdale, D.S., Goldberg, J. (1996). The expanded racial and ethnic codes in the Medicare data files: Their completeness of coverage and accuracy. *American Journal of Public Health* 86: 712–716.

LaVeist, T.A. (1994). Beyond dummy variables and sample selection: What health services researchers ought to know about race as a variable. *Health Services Research* 29(1): 1–16.

Lee, E. (1966). A theory of migration. *Demography* 3: 47–57.

Limerick, P.N. (1995). Peace initiative: Using Mormons to rethink culture and ethnicity in American history. *Journal of Mormon History* 21(2): 1–29.

Lorenz, K. (1940). Durch Domestikation verursachte Stöungen arteigenen Verhaltens, *Zeitschrift für Angewandte Psychologie und Characterkunde* 59: 68, 69. Quoted in W.H. Tucker. (1994). *The Science and Politics of Racial Research*. Urbana, Illinois: University of Illinois Press.

Mahoney, J., Arnold, R.C., Sterner, B.L., Harris, A., Zwally, M.R. (1944). Penicillin treatment of early syphilis II. *Journal of the American Medical Association* 126: 63–67.

Mangalam, J.J. *Human Migration: A Guide to Migration Literature in English 1955–1962*. Lexington, Kentucky: University of Kentucky.

Marín, G., Sabogal, F., Marín, B., Otero-Sabogal, R., Peréz-Stable, E.J. (1987). Development of a short acculturation scale for Hispanics. *Hispanic Journal of Behavioral Sciences* 9: 183–205.

Martin, E., DeMaio, T.J., Campanelli, P.C. (1990). Context effects for census measures of race and Hispanic origin. *Public Opinion Quarterly* 54: 551–566.

Massey, J. (1980). Using interviewer observed race and respondent reported race in the Health Interview Survey. *Proceedings of the American Statistical Association Meetings: Social Statistics Section* (pp. 425–428). Alexandria, Virginia: American Statistical Association.

McFee, M. (1968). The 150% man: A product of Blackfeet acculturation. *American Anthropologist* 70: 1096–1103.

McKenney, N.N., Bennett, C.E. (1994). Issues regarding data on race and ethnicity: The Census Bureau experience. *Public Health Reports* 109: 16–25.

McNeil, D.G. Jr. (1998). Like politics, all political correctness is local. *New York Times*, October 11: E11.

Melville, M.B. (1988). Hispanics: Race, class, or ethnicity? *Journal of Ethnic Studies* 16(1): 67–83.

Merton, R.K. (1972). Insiders and outsiders: A chapter in the sociology of knowledge (1972). In W. Sollors (Ed.), (1996). *Theories of Ethnicity: A Classical Reader* (pp. 325–369). New York: New York University Press.

Montagu, A. (1984). *Man's Most Dangerous Myth: The Fallacy of Race* (4th rev. ed.). Cleveland, Ohio: World.

Moore, J.E. (1933). *The Modern Treatment of Syphilis*. Baltimore, Maryland: Charles C. Thomas.

Nagel, J. (1994). Constructing ethnicity: Creating and recreating ethnic identity and culture. *Social Problems* 41: 152–176.

Nahirny, V.C., Fishman, J.A. (1965). American immigrant groups: Ethnic identification and the problem of generations. In W. Sollors (Ed.), (1996). *Theories of Ethnicity: A Classical Reader* (pp. 266–281). New York: New York University Press.

Navarro, M. (1997). Black and Cuban-American: Bias in 2 worlds. *New York Times*, Sept. 13: 7.

Noojin, R.O., Callaway, J.L., Flower, A.H. (1945). Favorable response to penicillin therapy in a case of treatment-resistant syphilis. *North Carolina Medical Journal*, January: 34–37.

Oetting, E.R. (1993). Orthogonal cultural identification: Theoretical links between cultural identification and substance use. In M. DelaRosa (Ed.), *Drug Abuse among Minority Youth: Methodological Issues and Recent Research Advances* (NIDA Research Monograph No. 130). Rockville, Maryland: National Institute on Drug Abuse.

Oetting, E.R., Beauvais, F. (1990). Orthogonal cultural identification theory: The cultural identification of minority adolescents. *International Journal of the Addictions* 25: 655–685.

Oetting, E.R., Swaim, R.C., Chairella, M.C. (1998). Factor structure and invariance of the Orthogonal Cultural Identification Scale among American Indian and Mexican American youth. *Hispanic Journal of Behavioral Sciences* 20(2): 131–154.

Olmedo, E.L., Martinez, J.L., Martinez, S.R. (1978). Measure of acculturation for Chicano adolescents. *Psychological Reports* 42: 159–170.

Olmedo, E.L., Padilla, A.M. (1978). Empirical and construct validation of a measure of acculturation for Mexican Americans. *Journal of Social Psychology* 105: 179–187.

Osborne, N.G., Feit, F.D. (1992). The use of race in medical research. *Journal of the American Medical Association* 267(2): 275–279.

Otero-Sabogal, R., Sabogal, F., Perez-Stable, E.J. (1995). Psychosocial correlates of smoking among immigrant Latina adolescents. *Journal of the National Cancer Institute Monograph* 18: 65–71.

Padilla, A.M. (1980). The role of cultural awareness and ethnic loyalty. In A.M. Padilla (Ed.), *Acculturation: Theory, Models and New Findings* (pp. 47–84). Boulder, Colorado: Westview Press.

Padilla, F. (1985). *Latino Ethnic Consciousness: The case of Mexican-Americans and Puerto Ricans in Chicago*. Notre Dame: University of Notre Dame Press.

Padilla, F. (1986). Latino ethnicity in the city of Chicago. In S. Olzak, J. Nagel (Eds.), *Competitive Ethnic Relations* (pp. 153–171). New York: Academic Press.

Pappas, G. (1993). *La Raza—Identify Yourselves!* Denver, Colorado: Latin American Research and Service Agency.

People v. Hall. (1854). 4 Cal. 399.

Pereira de Queiroz, M.I. (1986). Identite nationale, religion, expressions culturelles: La creation religieuse au Bresil [National identity, religion, cultural expression: Religious creation in Brazil]. *Information sur les Sciences Sociales* [*Information on Social Sciences*] 25: 207–227.

Personal Responsibility and Work Opportunity Reconciliation Act of 1996, Pub. L. No. 104–193, 110 Stat. 2105. August 11, 1996.

Pesare, P.J., Bauer, T.J., Gleeson, J.A. (1950). Untreated syphilis in the male Negro: Observation of abnormalities over sixteen years. *American Journal of Syphilis, Gonorrhea, and Venereal Diseases* 34: 201–213.

Pintner, R. (1923). *Intelligence Testing: Methods and Results.* New York: Henry Holt.

Quillian, D.D. (1906). Racial peculiarities: A cause of the prevalence of syphilis in Negroes. *American Journal of Dermatology & Genito-Urinary Disease* 10: 277–279.

Ramirez, M., III. (1984). Assessing and understanding biculturalism-multiculturalism in Mexican-American adults. In J.L. Martinez, R.H. Mendoza (Eds.), *Chicano Psychology* (pp. 325–345). New York: Academic Press.

Redfield, R., Linton, R., Herskovits, M.J. (1936). Memorandum on the study of acculturation. *American Anthropologist* 38: 149–152.

Resnicow, K., Soler, R.E., Braithwaite, R.L., Selassie, M.B., Smith, M. (1999). Development of a racial and ethnic identity scale for African American adolescents: The survey of black life. *Journal of Black Psychology* 25(2): 171–188.

Riddell-Heaney, J. (2003). Safeguarding children: 3. Getting to grips with culture and ethnicity. *Professional Nurse* 18(8): 473–475.

Rivers, E., Schuman, S.H., Simpson, L., Olansky, S. (1953). Twenty years of followup experience in a long-range medical study. *Public Health* Reports 68: 391–395.

Rose, A.M. (1956). Sociology: The Study of Human Relations. New York: Alfred A. Knopf.

Runciman, W.G. (Ed.). (1978). *Weber: Selections in Translation.* Cambridge: Cambridge University Press.

Russell, K., Wilson, M., Hall, R. (1992). *The Color Complex: The Politics of Skin Color among African Americans.* New York: Harcourt, Brace Jovanovich.

Sanjek, S. (1994). The enduring inequalities of race. In S. Gregory, R. Sanjek (Eds.), *Race* (pp. 1–17). New Brunswick, New Jersey: Rutgers University Press.

Sankar, P. (2003). MEDLINE definitions of race and ethnicity and their application to genetic research. *Nature Genetics* 34: 119.

Schiller, N.G., Crystal, S., Lewellen, D. (1994). Risky business: The cultural construction of AIDS risk groups. *Social Science & Medicine* 38: 1337–1346.

Segal, D.A. (1991). The European. *Anthropology Today* 7(5): 7–9.

Segen, J.C. (1992). *The Dictionary of Modern Medicine.* Park Ridge, New Jersey: Parthenon Publishing Group.

Siegel, J.S., Passel, J.S. (1979). *Coverage of the Hispanic Population of the United States in the 1970 Census.* Washington, D.C.: Bureau of the Census [Current Population Reports, United States Department of Commerce Pub. P23, No. 82].

Snipp, C.M. (1986). Who are American Indians? Some observations about the perils and pitfalls of data for race and ethnicity. *Population Research Policy Review* 5: 237–252.

Social Science Research Council. (1954). Acculturation: An exploratory formulation. *American Anthropologist* 56: 973–1002.

Stone, D.A. (1988). *Policy Paradox and Political Reason.* Boston: Little, Brown.

Stone, J., Dennis, R. (2003). Introduction: Race against time—the ethnic divide in the twentieth century. In J. Stone, R. Dennis (Eds.), *Race and Ethnicity: Comparative and Theoretical Approaches* (pp. 1–7). Malden, Massachusetts: Blackwell Publishing.

Thernstrom, S. (Ed.). (1980). *Harvard Encyclopedia of American Ethnic Groups.* Cambridge, Massachusetts: Belknap.

Thomas, S.B., Quinn, S.C. (1991). The Tuskegee syphilis study, 1932 to 1972: Implications for HIV education and AIDS risk education programs in the black community. *American Journal of Public Health* 81: 1498–1504.

Tucker, W.H. (1994). *The Science and Politics of Racial Research.* Urbana, Illinois: University of Illinois Press.

Velez-Ibáñez, C. (1996). *Border Visions.* Tucson, Arizona: University of Arizona Press.

Waters, M. (1990). *Ethnic Options: Choosing Identities in America.* Berkeley, California: University of California Press.

Williams, D.R., LaVizzo-Mourey, R., Warren, R.C. (1994). The concept of race and health status in America. *Public Health Reports* 109: 126–141.

Yanow, D. (2003). *Constructing "Race" and "Ethnicity" in America: Category-Making in Public Policy and Administration.* Armonk, New York: M.E. Sharpe.

Yinger, J.M. (1994). *Ethnicity: Source of Strength? Source of Conflict?* Albany, New York: State University of New York Press.

4
Defining Sex, Gender, and Sexual Orientation

Sex

It has generally been assumed that human beings must biologically be of either the male or female sex. Whether an individual is identified as a biological male or female is premised on an evaluation of chromosomal sex, gonadal sex, and morphological sex and secondary sex traits (Herdt, 1994). Lillie's thoughts on sexual dimorphism reflect this assumption that human *must* be either male or female:

What exists in nature is a dimorphism within species into male and female individuals, which differ with respect to contrasting characters, for each of which in any given species we recognize a male form and a female form, whether these characters be classed as of the biological, or psychological, or social orders. Sex is not a force that produces these contrasts; it is merely a name for our total impression of the differences... In the strictly historical sense of these words, a male is to be defined as an individual that produces spermatozoa; a female one that produces ova; or individuals at least having the characters associated with these functions (Lillie, 1939).

The sexologist John Money made similar assumptions regarding the dichotomous nature of sex and its relationship to gender. Kessler (1998) has asserted that five basic premises provided the foundation to Money's work: (1) genitals are naturally dimorphic; (2) genitals that blur this dimorphism require surgical correction; (3) gender is dichotomous because genitals are dimorphic; (4) dimorphic genitals serve as markers of dichotomous gender; and (5) medical professionals have legitimate authority to define the relationship between gender and genitals.

   In the usual course of events, the chromosomal sex of an embryo is determined by the fertilization of an ovum by either an X-bearing or a Y-bearing sperm. Fertilization by an X-bearing sperm results in an XX zygote, which normally develops into a female. In contrast, fertilization by a Y-bearing sperm produces an XY zygote, which normally develops into a male (Moore and Persaud, 1993). Prior to the seventh week of an embryo's development, however, the gonads of both males and females are identical in appearance and are therefore referred to as indifferent or undifferentiated gonads. Sexual differentiation of the gonads will occur during the first half of fetal life, as will the development of the internal genital tract and the external genitalia (Josso, 1981). Hormonal sex will emerge at puberty and may affect one's psychological sex (Josso, 1981). As will be seen in the discussion that follows, however, this process is not without variation.

Sexual Deviance

Variance from what has been considered the biological norm has often been as deviant, rather than a reflection of diversity (Brierley, 2000). The models that have been formulated to explain deviance are important in understanding the various approaches that have been adopted to explain and categorize sex, sexuality, and sexual behavior and, consequently, the issues that may arise in attempt to assess sex, gender, sexual orientation, and related constructs.

Brierley (2000) has identified five models of sexual deviance: the classificatory, psychodynamic, biological, sociological, and human rights models. Brierley uses the term "classificatory model" to label what others have referred to as the medical model. This model attempts to classify seemingly similar behaviors together into diagnostic categories of illnesses that require treatment or cure. The psychodynamic model utilizes a similar approach in that variation is perceived as perversion that requires a remedy, often psychotherapy, to rechannel sexual interests and desires. This approach has euphemistically been referred to as "change therapy," implying that any distress experienced by the individual as a result of his or her "condition" is attributable to his or her inability to engage in socially desirable behavior. Neither the classificatory nor the psychodynamic models admit the likelihood or even possibility that it is society that requires a change or cure, rather than the individual. The biological model similarly presumes that deviation from the norm requires "fixing," which can be effectuated through a variety of treatments that may include hormone therapy and surgery (Brierley, 2000).

Unlike the previously mentioned three models, the sociological and human rights models view the "problem" of "sexual deviance" as having been manufactured by the larger society. The sociological model focuses diversity of sexual behavior as a matter of statistical variation. The human rights model argues that by viewing sexual variation as deviance, society violates the rights of minority groups (Brierley, 2000).

Intersexuality, Hemaphroditism, and Pseudohermaphroditism

Discrepancy between the morphology of the gonads (testes or ovaries) and the appearance of the external genitalia results in intersexuality, also referred to as hermaphroditism. Although the terms are often used interchangeably, they embody differing perspectives about sexual ambiguity. Dreger (1998: 31) has explained:

"Intersexed" literally means that an individual is *between* the sexes—that s/he slips between and blends maleness and femaleness. By contrast the term "hermaphroditic" implies that a person has *both* male and female attributes, that s/he is not a third sex or a blended sex, but instead that s/he is a sort of double sex, that is, in possession of a body which juxtaposes essentially "male" and essentially "female" parts.

Not only have individuals been classified as hermaphrodites or intersex, but those that have, have been subject to further classification of their sexuality. The French surgeon Samuel Pozzi believed that one's sex was dependent on one's gonads (Dreger, 1998). He recommended during the early 20th century that hermaphrodites be classified as follows:

I. *Asexed or oligosexed.* Subjects indifferent or nearly indifferent from the sexual point of view.
II. *Homosexed or inverted.* Among these, we can admit a subdivision: In one category, the inversion appears very much to be a secondary effect of causes acting *artificially*, if we may say it this way, on the mentality and the habits of the subject [as though "mistaken" sexual education]. In another category, it seems that the inversion was original or innate.
III. *Heterosexed* or individuals having the sexual appetite directed toward women if they have testicles, toward men if they have ovaries. (It might be preferable ... to call them *orthosexed*, that is to say, sexed in the normal direction (Dreger, 1998: 129–130).

It is evident from this classification system that hermaphroditism both provoked significant confusion and was erroneously equated with sexual orientation. Some scholars, such as Jonathon Hutchinson, hypothesized in 1896 that sexual inversion [homosexuality] might be associated with overlooked or undetected hermaphroditic traits (Dreger, 1998). Ellis, a physician in London, posited:

It seems to me, on a review of all the facts that have come under my observation, that while there is no necessary connection between infantilism [the persistence of childish features], feminism ["feminine" features in a man], and masculinism ["masculine" features in a woman], physical and psychic, on the one hand, and sexual inversion on the other, yet there is a distinct tendency for the signs of the former group of abnormalities to occur with unusual frequency in inverts (Ellis, 1908: 171).

The analogy drawn between hermaphroditism and homosexuality permitted the inference that, like hermaphroditism, homosexuality, or inversion, was pathological and that intersex represented an inferior form of life because it existed between malehood and femalehood (Dreger, 1998). The consequences of this inference are discussed further in chapter 4.

In contrast, the teratologist Isidore Geoffroy Saint-Hilaire classified hermpahroditic individuals based on their possession of "excess" body parts. The first class, consisting of those individuals without excess body parts, were further classified into four orders based on the appearance of their sexual apparatus as essentially, female, male neuter, or mixed. The second class consisted of three orders: the complex masculine hermaphrodism [*sic*], which included individuals bearing male sexual apparatus and supernumerary female parts; the complex feminine hermaphrodism [*sic*], such that they had female sexual apparatus and supernumerary male parts; and bisexual hermpahrodism [*sic*], which referred to individuals with either complete male and female sexual apparatus or individuals in which one or both of the apparatuses were incomplete (Dreger, 1998). Other classification systems were also devised, including those of the obstetrician Simpson, who categorized hermpahroditism into spurious and true.

Today, the medical literature tends to speak of hermaphroditism as being classifiable into three distinct types: true hermaphroditism, male pseudohermaphroditism, and female pseudohermaphroditism (Dreger, 1998). True hermaphroditism is extremely rare and occurs only when both testicular and ovarian tissue are present. These tissues, however, are generally nonfunctional (Krob, Braun, and Kuhnle, 1994; Moore and Persaud, 1993; Talerman, Verp, Senekjian, Gilewski, and Vogelzang, 1990). The majority of true hermaphrodites appear to have an XX chromosomal basis, although some may have XY chromosomes and others exhibit chimerism, whereby some cells display XX chromosomes and others exhibit XY chromosomes. It is believed that chimerism occurs as the result of the fusion of two early embryos, one XX and one XY, into one individual. The genitalia of true hermaphrodites may appear "typically" male or female, or may appear otherwise (Dreger, 1998).

Approximately one-half of all instances of ambiguous external genitalia are believed to be individuals with female pseudohermaphroditism (Moore, 1989). Female pseudohermaphroditism is characterized by the existence of ovaries and an XX chromosomal basis. As the result of exposure to high levels of the hormone androgen while in the womb, the external genitalia of these individuals appear masculinized, so that what is assumed to be the clitoris may look and act like a penis, and what is assumed to be the labia may resemble a scrotum. However, the internal organs appear to be those of a biological female.

There have been various theories advanced in an attempt to understand and explain the masculinization of female pseudohermaphroditism. It has been suggested that a tumor on the suprarenal gland of the pregnant mother could result in the excessive production of androgens, thereby effecting a "male" type development of the female child's genitalia. Alternatively, masculinization of a female child could result from the administration of androgenic hormones to a pregnant women, for instance, in order to prevent a miscarriage. Finally, congenital adrenal hyperplasia, or CAH, may be responsible for the masculinization of a female child, through the production of large amounts of androgens by the adrenal glands. Although the fetus has an XX chromosomal basis and ovaries, the increased amount of androgens may result in the development of external genitalia associated with males (Moore, 1989; Thompson, McInnes, and Willard, 1991). The prevalence of this condition has been estimated to be anywhere from 1 in 12,500 births to 1 in every 60,000 births (Dreger, 1998).

Male pseudohermaphroditism may result from two or more causes. Individuals with androgen insensitivity syndrome (AIS) have an XY chromosome basis and testes but are unable to respond to testosterone produced by the testes as the result of an androgen receptor defect (Groveman, 1999). The androgen insensitivity may be partial or complete (Mignon, Brown, and Fichman, 1981). As a result of this deficiency, the genitals may appear to be those of a female and the secondary sex characteristics may also be those of a female. Researchers have estimated that approximately 1 out of every 120,000 individuals have AIS (Jagiello and Atwell, 1962). Many individuals with AIS may not know that they have this condition until they seek medical advice during puberty because of their failure to menstruate (Dreger, 1998).

Male pseudohermaphroditism may also result from a condition known as 5-alpha-reductase (5-AR) deficiency. These individuals are genetically and gonadally male, but as a result of this condition, their external genitalia appear feminine at birth (Wilson and Reiner, 1999). The enzyme 5-alpha-reductase is critical to the conversion of testosterone to dihydrotestosterone. Although the testes of the child produce testosterone during fetal development, the testosterone is not converted due to the deficiency of this enzyme. As a result, the fetus develops genitalia that appear to be those of a female. However, additional testosterone is produced by the testes at puberty; this testosterone is adequate to produce "masculine" features because the enzyme is not required to process the testosterone at puberty. Individuals with this condition may develop facial hair, the testes may descend, and what was believed to be a clitoris may grow and look more like a penis (Wilson, 1992).

Ambiguous genitalia may also result from a number of other conditions, such as Klinefelter's syndrome and Turner's syndrome (Wilson and Reiner, 1999). In Klinefelter's syndrome, the male child has an XXY chromosomal basis, while in Turner's syndrome, a girl is missing all or part of her second X chromosome.

Ultimately, what is considered to be hemaphroditism or ambiguous sex will depend in any given context on what is accepted within a given culture and context as a normal variation of maleness/malehood or femaleness/femalehood and what is considered to be truly ambiguous. This, in turn, requires the identification of the characteristics that are believed to be critical to the status of malehood and femalehood. Kessler (1998) has argued for the characterization of intersexuality as a reflection of variability, rather than ambiguity. Genitals that vary in form from a predetermined standard may embody a number of different meanings: (1) the genitals do not reflect either of the two traditional gender categories and testing is consequently warranted; (2) the genitals reflect the "wrong" gender category, therefore necessitating surgical correction; (3) the genitals do not conform to the known gender but will correct themselves; (4) the nonconforming genitals are indicative of an underlying medical condition that requires nonsurgical intervention; (5) the genitals are inferior and require surgical correction; (6) the genitals are superior and are the object of envy; (7) the genitals vary from person to person; or (8) the nature of one's genitals reflects the misbehavior or genetic unsuitability of his or her parents. Just as the meaning that attaches to "ambiguity" varies over time and place, so too may the interpretation given to perceived variability. Indeed, "variability" can only be perceived in reference to a predetermined standard of desirability and/or normality.

The Intersex Society of North America (ISNA) seeks the cessation of all intersex-related surgery until an individual can consent for him- or herself. ISNA has argued that intersex surgeries are more appropriately termed "intersex genital mutilation," or IGM, in a manner analogous to ritualized cutting of female genitalia, also known as female genital mutilation (FGM) and female circumcision (Kessler, 1998).

Gender, Gender Role, and Gender Identity

Gender and Gender Role

Traditionally, one's biological sex has been linked to one's gender, gender role, and social identity. One scholar observed this seemingly inextricable linkage of the two concepts with the following example:

[W]omen's low brain weights and deficient brain structures were analogous to those of lower races, and their inferior intellectualities explained on this basis. Women, it was observed, shared with Negroes a narrow, childlike, and delicate skull, so different from the more robust and rounded heads characteristics of males of "superior" races. Similarly, women of higher races tended to have slightly protruding jaws, analogous to, if not exaggerated as, the apelike jutting jaws of lower races. Women and lower races were called innately impulsive, emotional, imitative rather than original, and incapable of the abstract reasoning found in white men (Stepan, 1990: 39–40).

Stoller distinguished the concepts of sex and gender, arguing that sex is a function of biology, while gender is a function of culture:

Dictionaries stress that the major connotation of sex is a biological one as, for example, in the phrases *sexual relations* or the *male sex* . . . . It is for some of these psychological phenomena [behavior, feelings, thoughts, fantasies] that the term *gender* will be used: one can speak of the male sex or the female sex but one can also talk about masculinity or femininity and not necessarily be implying anything about anatomy or physiology (Stoller, 1968: viii–ix).

However, Stoller also appears to rely on biology in defining gender when referring to normality of masculinity and femininity:

Gender is a term that has psychological and cultural rather than biological connotations; if the proper terms for sex are "male" and "female," the proper terms for gender are "masculine" and "feminine"; the latter may be quite independent of (biological) sex. Gender is the amount of masculinity or femininity found in a person and, obviously, while there are mixtures of both in many humans, the *normal* male has a preponderance of masculinity and the *normal* female a preponderance of femininity. (Emphasis added.)

In contrast, gender has been defined as

a multidimensional category of personhood encompassing a distinct pattern of social and cultural differences. Gender categories often draw on perceptions of anatomical and physiological differences between bodies, but those perceptions are always mediated by cultural categories and meanings . . . . Gender categories are not only "models of" difference . . . but also "models for" difference. They convey gender-specific expectations for behavior and temperament, sexuality, kinship and interpersonal roles, occupation, religious roles and other social patterns. Gender categories are "total social phenomena" . . . .; a wide range of institutions and beliefs find simultaneous expression through them, a characteristic that distinguishes gender from other social statuses (Roscoe, 1994: 341).

Yet another scholar explained:

Gender is a way in which social practice is ordered. In gender processes, the everyday conduct of life is organized in relation to a reproductive arena, define by bodily structures and processes of human reproduction. This arena includes sexual arousal and intercourse, childbirth and infant care, bodily sex difference and similarity.

I call this a 'reproductive arena' not a 'biological base' to emphasize the point... that we are talking about a historical process involving the body, not a fixed set of biological determinants. Gender is a social practice that constantly refers to bodies and what bodies do, it is not a social practice reduced to the body ... Gender exists precisely to the extent that biology does *not* determine the social. It marks one of those points of transition where the historical process supersedes biological evolution as the form of change (Connell, 2005: 71).

Gender role, then, is

[e]verything that a person says and does, to indicate to others or to the self the degree that one is either male, or female, or ambivalent; it includes but is not restricted to sexual arousal and response (Money and Erhardt, 1972).

The adoption of a "male" style of dress and behavior by "sworn virgins" of northern Albania serves to illustrate how specific behaviors and other social patterns are associated with a specific gender and reflected in gender role. The "sworn virgins" vow to become men and dress and behave in a manner consonant with the societal expectations of men (Young, 2000). Several motives have been identified for this course of action:

In traditional Albanian society there is no such sophisticated (and expensive) surgical assistance for social and psychological transition. However, the reasons for the female-to-male cross gender role taken on by the women... have less to do with the individual than the social, economic, and cultural situation into which they are born. Early records refer predominantly to this as the only acceptable alternative to not marrying the man to whom a woman was betrothed. Another strong reason to encourage the change of gender is in order to become eligible to become a family head and a legal heir—an essential role to be filled in every family. Lack of a son of sufficient age and integrity (representing honour for a family) may bring shame... In order to cross the boundary from a woman's world to a man's domain, it is necessary to change sex socially: this is done by dressing as a man and socially engaging in activities limited to men (Young, 2000: 57).

As yet another example, we may consider the "mainstream" conceptualization of male and female gender and gender roles in the United States. Defining a "man," apart from a biological definition that incorporates hormone levels, chromosomes, and genital organs, is inextricably linked to our definition of "masculinity" (Whitehead and Barrett, 2001). "Masculinities" have been defined as

those behaviours, languages and practices, existing in specific cultural and organizational locations, which are commonly associated with males and thus culturally defined as not feminine. So masculinities exist as both a positive, inasmuch as they offer some means of identity signification for males, and as a negative, inasmuch as they are not the 'Other' (feminine) (Whitehead and Barrett, 2001: 15–16).

Seemingly, however, maleness and masculinity do not come naturally. Badinter (1995: 1–2) observed:

The order so often heard—"Be a man"—implies that it does not go without saying and that manliness may not be as natural as one would like to think. At the very least, the exhortation signifies that the possession of a Y chromosome or male sex organs is not enough to define the human male. Being a man implies a labor, an effort that does not seem to be demanded of a woman....Without being aware of it, we behave as though femininity were natural, therefore unavoidable, whereas masculinity must be acquired, and at a high price. The man himself and those who surround him are so unsure of his sexual identity that proofs of his manliness are required... Yet the display of proofs requires trials that a woman does not have to undergo. The day of her first period comes naturally, without effort if not without pain, and now the little girl is declared a woman forever. There is nothing like this, nowadays, for a little boy belonging to Western civilization.

The more positive traits associated with masculinity include a willingness to sacrifice self for family; loyalty, dedication, and commitment; the ability to solve problems and the willingness to take risks to do so; and self-reliance, fortitude, persistence, and calm (Levant, 1995). And, although conceptions of masculinity vary across different American subgroups, is has been asserted that

there is a core which is common to most: courage, endurance and toughness, lack of squeamishness when confronted with shocking or distasteful stimuli, avoidance of display in weakness in general, reticence about emotional or idealistic matters, and sexual competency (Stouffer, Lumsdaine, Lumsdaine et al., 1976).

Manhood in the United States, then, has been defined through various restrictive, societally-imposed edicts:

1. "No Sissy Stuff." One may never do anything that even remotely suggests femininity. Masculinity is the relentless repudiation of the feminine.
2. "Be a Big Wheel." Masculinity is measured by power, success, health, and status. As the saying goes, "He who has the most toys wins when he dies."
3. "Be a Sturdy Oak." Masculinity depends on remaining calm and reliable in crises, holding emotions in check. In fact, proving you're a man depends on never showing your emotions at all. Boys don't cry.
4. "Give 'em Hell." Exude an aura of manly daring and aggression. Go for it. Take risks. (Brannon, 1976).

Similarly, the "masculine mystique" emphasizes restrictive emotionality, health care problems, obsession with achievement and success, restricted sexual and affectionate behavior, and concerns about power, control, competition, and homophobia (O'Neil, 1982). The "elements" of the male role have been said to include "the anti-feminine element," the "success element," the "aggressiveness elements," and the "sexual element" (Doyle, 1989).

It has been argued that, as a consequence, the birthright of every American male is a chronic sense of personal inadequacy (Woolfolk and Richardson, 1978) and that men's true fear "is not fear of women but of being ashamed or humiliated in front of other men, or being dominated by stronger men" (Leverenz, 1986: 451). If this is, indeed, true, then homophobia has little to do with homosexual experience and everything to do with, as one man stated,

the fear that other men will unmask us, emasculate us, reveal to us and the world that we do not measure up, that we are not real men. We are afraid to let other men see that fear. Fear makes us ashamed, because the recognition of fear in ourselves is proof to ourselves that we are not as manly as we pretend.... (Kimmel, 2003: 104).

It has been hypothesized that, as a result, the development of male gender identity involves the construction of positional identities, whereby a sense of the self is solidified through separation from others (Chodorow, 1978). This stands in sharp contrast to the development of female gender identity, which often involves the definition of self through one's connections with others (Gilligan, 1982). For men who both fear and desire connection with others, organized sports provides a mechanism for interaction, while still focusing on hierarchical position, e.g., being number one (Messner, 2003).

The establishment of positional identity is evident in other domains, as well. One psychiatrist commented:

Men become depressed because of loss of status and power in the world of men. It is not the loss of money, or the material advantages that money could buy, which produces the despair that leads to self-destruction. It is the "shame," the "humiliation," the sense of personal "failure".... A man despairs when he has ceased being a man among men (Gaylin, 1992: 32).

Accordingly, this process of establishing and asserting one's identity is said, then, to explain much of heterosexual male behavior in the United States: men must act in a way that eliminates any possibility that others will get the "wrong idea": withholding any expression of feelings, displaying sexual predation with women, walking and talking in a specified manner (Kimmel, 2003). There are, however, exceptional situations in which men are permitted to behave in ways that, under other circumstances, would negate their masculinity. Depictions of war, for instance, allow men to hold and comfort each other (Easthope, 1986).

It has been argued, though, that the establishment of a male identity has become increasingly difficult for men due to relatively recent profound changes in men's situations: women's increasing exercise of choice in relationships, divorce, and child-bearing; the decreasing likelihood that men will enjoy a secure, life-long career or employment situation; the increasing number of dual-income households in lieu of households where the male is the sole breadwinner; and the increasing visibility of groups once relegated to society's margins, such as gay men, women, and persons of color (Whitehead and Barrett, 2001).

Violence, it has been asserted, or the willingness to engage in violence, constitutes one mechanism for the establishment of manhood and masculinity or, in other words, positional identity (Gilligan, 2001; Kimmel, 2003). This is reflected in the observation that the insults most shaming to men are those that challenge the existence or the extent of their courage or manliness, including their sexual adequacy: "wimp," "coward," "sissy," "fairy" (Gilligan, 2001: 571). One writer observed:

Little boys learn the connection between violence and manhood very early in life. Fathers indulge in mock prize fights and wrestling matches with eight-year-olds. Boys play cowboys and Indians with guns and arrows proffered by their elders. They are gangsters or soldiers interchangeably—the lack of difference between the two is more evident to them than to their parents. They are encouraged to "fight back," and bloodied noses and black eyes become trophies of their pint-sized virility (Komisar, 1976).

In contrast to men, women are shamed by insults that allude to their being too much like men: too independent, too aggressive; transposed into a sexual context, this becomes a "bitch," "whore," "tramp," or "slut." Not surprisingly, in a survey of both men and women, men expressed their greatest fear as being laughed at. In contrast, women's greatest fear was of being raped and murdered (Noble, 1992). It is of note that the term "cuckhold," meaning an inability to control one's partner's sexuality, is applied exclusively to men, whereas the term "promiscuous" is used almost exclusively to refer to women's behavior (Gilligan, 2001).

Exclusionary devices offer an additional route for the establishment and maintenance of a positional hierarchy. Through exclusion, those deemed less manly are relegated to lower positions in the hierarchy—women, gay men, men of color, non-native-born men, men of lower socioeconomic status. Those men deemed to be less "manly" reflect subordinate and marginal masculinities (Whitehead and Barrett, 2001). Through exclusion, "manhood" embodies sexism, racism, and homophobia (Kimmel, 2003).

Notman (1982: 4) has explained that "Femininity is very difficult to define because the word is used in a number of ways. It can be used descriptively, normatively, diagnostically, clinically, and colloquially." Early concepts of femininity, such as those espoused by Freud and Deutsch, consisted of a triad of characteristics: passivity, masochism, and narcissism (Deutsch, 1944, 1945; Freud, 1961). More recent psychoanalytic thought has been careful to distinguish between gender identity, gender role, and the qualities of masculinity and femininity (Notman, 1982).

In contrast to this psychoanalytic perspective, Bartky (1990: 65) has argued that

We are born male or female, but not masculine or feminine. Femininity is an artifice, an achievement, 'a mode of enacting and reenacting received gender norms which surface as so many styles of the flesh' (quoting Butler, 1985: 11).

Femininity, according to Jay (1981) has been said to represent the not-masculinity, the not-A. This view has been reflected in popularly marketed literature. For instance, a 1948 book explained to teen-age girls that "*the normal boy is attracted to the completely feminine girl*" and the "normal girl" likes "*a man who is completely masculine, the direct opposite of you*" (Bryant, 1948, emphasis in original).

The ideal depiction of the feminine girl was represented at one time by the figure of Jane in the dyad of Dick and Jane, the characters who first appeared in all of the stories in the 1930 Elson Basic reader pre-primer. It has been estimated that by 1950, 80% of all first-graders in the United States were learning to read by growing up with Dick and Jane (Kismaric and Heiferman, 1996).

Dick of Dick and Jane embodied the ideal of the all-American boy: confident, direct, responsible, organized, in control, resourceful, and well-behaved. Jane, on the other hand, never quite measured up to the same standard. She has something new to wear on every page; in fact, her dresses never wrinkled and never dirtied. Jane never sulked and never lost her temper. Her hair was not too curly, but not too straight; Jane was not too fat, but not too thin. Jane reflected what girls should be: "The ideal middle-class girl of the 1950s was ladylike and wore dresses everywhere, accessorized with hats, shoes, purses and clean white gloves to create a total 'look'" (Kismaric and Heiferman, 1996: 26). While Dick was a character of substance, with real personality and strength, Jane was a superficial soul, delighted to look pretty and look wistfully on while Dick accomplished his successes. Little Sally, the baby of the family, depicted yet another aspect of the feminine: the doll baby who was always active, unthinkingly creating difficulties, and making people laugh with her antics. Jane and Sally were both blondes, unlike Dick, who was dark-haired.

Mother of the Dick and Jane series reflected similar features. Mother was blond, pretty, a good partner to Father, a nurturer of the children and her husband, an effortless homemaker. Mother likes to look good and "dresses like a lady" in pretty dresses (even while doing housework) and has matching pocketbooks. Mother always remembered to sit with her ankles crossed and her hands clasped. According to some writers, she does not work outside of the home, because her place is in the home, making sure that everything is always in its rightful place (Havemann and West, 1952). In fact, careers would lead to the

masculinization of women with enormously dangerous consequences to the home, the children dependent on it and to the ability of the woman, as well as her husband, to obtain sexual gratification (Friedan, 1963: 42, quoting Farnham and Lundberg).

Instead, Mother is selfless and soothing, dedicating her life to her family (Kismaric and Heiferman, 1996). As late as the 1960s, women's magazines encouraged their readers to assume such characteristics:

Psychiatrists call this characteristic "essential feminine altruism." Simply stated, it means that the hallmark of real femininity is...regard for and devotion to the interests of others...For the true woman, then, children and husband come first, way before self, for that is how her altruism expresses itself (Robinson, 1960: 62).

At least through the 1950s, the popular U.S. conceptualization of femininity sometimes appeared to minimize or negate the possession of intelligence or education. The Jungian analyst Mrs. Florida Scott-Maxwell (1958: 156) counseled her readers in *Ladies' Home Journal*:

When a woman begins to understand herself, she understands she has a masculine side as well as a feminine side and that masculine side is in constant danger of getting out of hand in our industrial, emancipated society. When a girl is in college and cultivates her mind, this may stimulate, even inflate, the masculine side, and she can become aridly intellectual, with a strong power drive, and then it is easy to become a doctor or a lawyer who is hardly feminine at all.

According to other writers, however, such as Duvall and Hill (1947: 210), some women risked their marriages if they failed to work:

Some women are temperamentally so built that if they do not have a job of their own they either "blow up" or constantly meddle in the affairs of their husbands, and possibly those of other husbands as well. With them a real job outside of the office meets a vital psychological need.

Women working in the office were counseled to be feminine and not just female:

Your over-all appearance should be such that the people with whom you are working will be aware of the fact that you are feminine, not just female... To be "female" at the office is a nuisance and therefore a waste of after-hours attractions (Ludden, 1956: 166).

Jane, like Dick and the world that they lived in, was entirely white. It was not until 1965 that non-white characters appeared to inhabit Dick and Jane's idyllic world. For over 30 years, "femininity" had been defined for school-aged children as applying to white girls and women only.

Femininity has also been equated with a particular body build or image. For instance, columnist Dolly Martin wrote in 1964, in seeming surprise, that "It's hard to picture a girl of large build being quite feminine, yet many chubby girls have very pleasing tendencies" (Martin, 1964: 8). Bartky (1990) has asserted that the construction of a "feminine" body from a female one, that is, the aesthetic of femininity, demands fragility and a lack of muscular strength, resulting in the inability to defend oneself physically; smooth and hairless skin, thereby infantilizing the body of grown women; and body language that is reflective of both tension and constriction. Ultimately, Bartky argues, women's adherence to this "performance" may engender attention, but affords little respect or social power and serves to demean everything that is female. In fact, women's attempts to adhere to an externally-imposed construction of femininity actually results in the diminution of women specifically because of this focus on what could be considered trivialities, such as body image. Bartky (1990: 80) maintains that the

woman who checks her make-up half a dozen times a day to see if her foundation has caked or her mascara run, who worries that the wind or rain may spoil her hairdo, who looks frequently to see if her stockings have bagged at the ankle, or who, feeling fat, monitors everything she eats, has become... a self-policing object, a self committed to a relentless self-surveillance. This self-surveillance is a form of obedience to patriarchy.

Gender Identity and Sexual Identity

Gender identity and gender role are also distinct concepts:

Gender identity has been defined as the private experience of gender role: the experience of one's sameness, unity and the persistence of one's individuality as male, female, or androgynous, expressed in both self-awareness and in behavior. Gender role is everything that a person says and does to indicate to others or to the self the degree to which one is either male, female or androgynous. Gender role would thus include public presentations of self in dress and verbal and nonverbal communication; the economic and family roles one plays; the sexual feelings (desires) one has and the persons to whom such feelings are directed; the sexual role one plays and emotions one experiences and displays; and the experiencing of one's body, as it is defined as masculine or feminine in any particular society. Gender identity and gender role are said to have a unity, like two sides of a coin (Nanda, 1994: 395–396).

Money and Erhardt (1972) similarly distinguished between the concept of gender and that of gender identity:

Gender Identity: The sameness, unity, and persistence of one's individuality as male, female, or ambivalent, in greater or lesser degree, especially as it is experienced in self awareness and behaviour; gender identity is the private experience of gender role, and gender role is the public expression of gender identity.

Stoller also discusses gender identity and gender role as they relate to the public-private distinction:

I am using the word *identity* to mean one's own awareness (whether one is conscious of it or not) of one's existence or purpose in this world or, to put it a bit differently, the organization of those psychic components that are to preserve one's awareness of existing (Stoller, 1968: x).

The concept of gender identity is also distinguishable from that of core gender identity, which represents a "person's unquestioning certainty that he belongs to one of only two sexes" (Stoller, 1968: 39):

This essentially unalterable core of gender identity [I am a male] is to be distinguished from the related but different belief, I am manly (or masculine). The latter attitude is a more subtle and complicated development. It emerges only after a child learned how his parents expect him to express masculinity (Stoller, 1968: 40).

In contrast to core gender identity, which signifies the feeling that "I am a male" or "I am a female," gender role represents "a masculine or feminine way of behaving" (Walinder, 1967: 74). The concept of sexual identity is also distinct, in that it

is ambiguous, since it may refer to one's sexual activities or fantasies, etc. . . . Thus, of a patient who says "I am not a very masculine man," it is possible to say that his gender identity is male although he recognizes his lack of so-called masculinity (Stoller, 1964: 220).

Transsexuality and Transgenderism

Transsexuality

The term *transsexual* has been used to refer to "individuals with a cross-sex identity," regardless of their surgical status or apparent biological sex (Bolin, 1992: 14). The fourth edition of the *Diagnosis and Statistical Manual* of the American

Psychiatric Association classified transsexuality as a gender identity disorder resulting in "clinically significant distress or impairment in social, occupational, or other important areas of functioning" (Reid and Wise, 1995: 241). Diagnosis of the "disorder" was premised on the existence of a "strong and persistent cross-gender identification" and "a persistent discomfort with one's sex or a sense of inappropriateness in the gender role of that sex" (Reid and Wise, 1995: 241). In addition, a diagnostic finding of transsexuality required differentiation from hermaphroditism, from a desire to change sex due to nonconformity with prescribed sexual roles, and from a desire to change sex to achieve a social or cultural advantage (Reid and Wise, 1995: 240). The current edition of the *Diagnostic and Statistical Manual, DSM-IV-Text Revision*, subsumes transsexuality within the classification of gender identity disorders (American Psychiatric Association, 2000). Table 3 indicates the basis for such a diagnosis in both children and adults.

It has been estimated that 1 out of every 11,900 men (male to female) and 1 out of every 30,400 women (female to male) are transsexual (Bakker, van Kesteren, Gooren, and Bezemer, 1993). Estimates of the male-female sex ratio have varied widely, ranging from 2.5 to 1 in the Netherlands to 5.5 to 1 in Poland (Bakker et al., 1993; Godlewski, 1988; Pauley, 1968).

Treatment for transsexualism has often consisted of long-term hormonal therapy and sex change surgery. Genital reassignment surgery from female to male is complex and extensive, requiring several stages to be completed (Hage, Bouman, de Graaf, and Bloem, 1993). Phalloplasty is used to construct a penis for female-to-male transsexuals (Hage, Bloem, and Suliman, 1993). Female-to male transsexuals often adhere to a long-term regimen of androgen administration in addition to undergoing surgery (Sapino, Pietribiasi, Godano, and Bussolati, 1992). Potential adverse outcomes may include necrosis, hernia, venous congestion, and phallic shaft fistulas (Hage, Bloem, and Suliman, 1993).

Male-to-female transsexuals wishing to modify their genitalia must also undergo extensive surgery (Eldh, 1993) and hormonal treatment (Valenta, Elias, and Domurat, 1992). Potential adverse outcomes include the lack of a sensate clitoris (Eldh, 1993), vaginal stenosis (Crichton, 1992; Stein, Tiefer, and Melman, 1990), and pain during sexual intercourse (Stein et al., 1990). The transition from male to female may also be emotionally stressful and difficult (Ames, 2005; Brevard, 2001; Griggs, 2004; Just Evelyn, 1998; Martino, 1977).

Many transsexual individuals may decide to forego surgery due to its high cost and lack of insurance coverage for such procedures (Gordon, 1991; Stein et al., 199) and the fear of an unsatisfactory surgical outcome (Crichton, 1992; Hage, Blout, Bloem, and Megens, 1993).

Transgenderism

The term *transgender* can be used to refer to (1) all those "who challenge the boundaries of sex and gender (Feinberg, 1996: x), (2) those who modify their sex with which they were labeled or identified with at birth, and (3) those individuals whose expressed gender is considered inappropriate for their apparent sex (Feinberg,

TABLE 3. Diagnostic criteria and symptoms for gender identity disorders

Diagnostic criterion	Symptoms exhibited by children	Symptoms exhibited by adults
Strong and persistent cross-gender identification	Four of the following:	Stated desire to be of the opposite sex
	Consistent statements that he or she is a member of the other sex or wishes to be a member of the opposite sex	Passing frequently as a member of the opposite sex
	Boys' preference for cross-dressing or girls' insistence on wearing stereotypical masculine clothes	A wish to live or be treated as a member of the opposite sex
	An assumption of cross-sex roles in make-believe play or persistent fantasy of being of the opposite sex	Believing that he or she has the feelings of a member of the opposite sex
	A strong wish to participate in games that are stereotypical of the opposite sex	
	A strong preference to have playmates of the opposite sex	
Persistent discomfort with his/her sex or a sense that the gender role of that sex is inappropriate	Boys: revulsion with penis, wish that it would fall off, rejection of games and toys typically associated with boys	Focus on attempting to eliminate primary and secondary sex characteristics
	Girls: stated desire to grow a penis and not to have breasts or menstruate	Belief that he/she was born a member of the wrong sex
Disturbance does not co-occur with a physical intersex condition		
Disturbance causes "clinically significant distress or impairment in social, occupational, or other important areas of functioning"		

Adapted from American Psychiatric Association (2000).

1996). Transgender individuals may be distinguished from transsexuals, who change or modify the sex that they were assigned at birth; in contrast to transsexuals, transgender individuals have been defined as those who "blur the [boundaries] of the *gender expression*" that is traditionally associated with the biological sexes (Feinberg, 1996). It has been asserted that "the guide principle of this [transgender] movement is that people should be free to change, either temporarily or permanently, the sex type to which they were assigned since infancy" (Rothblatt, 1995: 16).

Cross-dressing represents one such form of blurring (Garber, 1992). Cross-dressing, or wearing the clothing that is most frequently associated with the opposite biological sex, occurs for various reasons in numerous contexts; in fact, it may not be associated with transgenderism, depending upon its purpose and the context in which it occurs. Women may assume "an imitation man look" in order to succeed in business (Molloy, 1977). Males, regardless of their sexual orientation, may don women's clothing to perform as female impersonators. Gay men may cross-dress as a means of self-assertion or activism (Garber, 1992). Cross-dressing has been central in theater (Baker, 1994; Heriot, 1975) and, to a lesser degree, in religion (Barrett, 1931; Garber, 1992; Warner, 1982).

Sexual Orientation

Choosing a Sexual Partner: Sexual Attraction, Sexual Activity, and Self-Identity

In contrast to the term "heterosexuality," for which relatively few synonyms are used, homosexuality has been known by a vast number of other terms. These include uranianism, homogenic love, contrasexuality, homo-erotism, similsexualism, tribadism, sexual inversion, intersexuality, transexuality, third sex, and psychosexual hermaphroditism (Sell, 1997).

The apparent sex of one's sexual or romantic partner is often equated with one's sexual orientation. However, data indicate that homosexuality and homosexual behavior are not synonymous. One study of male sexual behavior in the United States found that 2% of the respondents ages 20 to 39 reported having had any same-sex sexual activity during the preceding 10 years, but only 1% reported exclusively same-sex sexual activity during the same time period (Billy, Tanfer, Grady, and Keplinger, 1993). An ethnographic study of men having sex with men found that only 14% of the individuals were primarily interested in homosexual relationships, over one-half of the men were married, and many of the married men engaged in sex with other men due to family planning concerns stemming from their observance of Catholic tenets relating to birth control (Humphreys, 1970). Identical sexual acts, including the choice of one's sexual partner, may vary in meaning and significance depending upon the cultural and historical context of the activities (Vance, 1995).

Homosexual behavior, as distinct from homosexuality, may reflect differentials in power and status between the partners. For instance, individuals may agree to participate in sex with an individual of the same sex in order to avoid the threat of increased violence; such situations are not uncommon in the context of living on the street (Scacco, 1992), imprisonment, and during war (Greenberg, 1988; Trexler, 1995).

In a number of societies, sexual relations between younger and older men were structured by age (Greenberg, 1988). The older male often assumed the active role in a relationship, while the younger male assumed the passive role. The sexual act could include masturbation, anal intercourse, and/or fellatio. The motivation for these relationships varied depending on the culture, but could derive from the belief that the older male could transmit special healing powers to the younger male through these acts; that physical maturation of the younger male required the implantation of semen in his body by an older adult; and/or that heterosexual intercourse would deplete one's vitality and/or harm men as a result of women's polluting qualities (Greenberg, 1988). Additionally, sex with other men may be a means of satisfying one's sexual needs in the absence of an adequate number of women.

The status of Native American berdache and Asian Indian hijra have often mistakenly been equated with homosexuality. A berdache has been defined as "a morphological male who does not fit society's standard man's role, who has a nonmasculine character" (Williams, 1992: 2). Native Americans often referred to berdaches as "halfmen-halfwomen," although they were neither transsexuals nore hermaphrodites. Berdaches, now more commonly referred to as "two-spirit people" (Lang, 1996), existed within a number of Native American tribes, including the Cheyenne, Creek, Klamath, Mohave, Navaho, Pima, Sioux, and Zuni (Greenberg, 1988; Roscoe, 1991; Williams, 1992). Two-spirit people have been described as androgynous and have been perceived as being of an alternative gender due to their use of the behaviors, social roles, and dress of both men and women. Although some individuals assumed the passive/receptive role in a sexual relationship with another man, the sexual relationship was a secondary component of one's status as a berdache (Callender and Kochens, 1985; Williams, 1992). Similarly, some two-spirit women adopted some male roles and dress and had sexual relations with women (Schaeffer, 1965). The berdache tradition, however, has declined due to missionary and U.S. government efforts. Additionally, younger Native Americans may have rejected the role of the berdache and self-identify, instead, as gay males (Williams, 1992).

The hijras of India have been called "neither man nor woman and woman and man" (Nanda, 1990, 1994). In the past, hijras have played a religious role, derived from Hinduism, by blessing newborn male children and performing at wedding ceremonies (Nanda, 1990). Hijras are defined as such by their lack of sexual desire for and sexual impotence with women, rather than by their sexual relations with men. Their impotence with women has been attributed to a defect in or absence of male sexual organs from birth or through their surgical removal (Nanda, 1990). Hijras self-define as "not men" due to their impotence with women and as "not women" because of their inability to bear children; as such, they collapse sex and gender into one category. They incorporate various aspects of the female role, such as dress, gendered erotic fantasies, a desire for male sexual partner, and a gender identity of a woman or hijra, with those of a male role, which include coarse speech and the use of the hookah for smoking (Nanda, 1994). Despite their sexual relations with other men, hijras do not self-define as homosexuals.

Sexual Orientation

The identification of an individual's sexual orientation is quite complex. The behavioral view of sexual orientation asserts that one determines sexual orientation by reference to the sex of the individual with whom one is involved sexually: if it is an individual of the same sex, then one is a homosexual, while if the person is of the opposite sex, one is heterosexual (Stein, 1999). However, this viewpoint suffers from a number of limitations. First, it equates behavior with orientation, despite the possibility that there may be multiple explanations for the same behaviors. Second, it assumes that only two sexual orientations exist. Third, the theory is concerned with whether the sexual partner is of the same or opposite sex, rather than whether the sexual partner is a man or woman. Additionally, it is unclear as to the exact point in time at which this assessment is to be made: Is it premised on the sex of the first person with whom one has sexual relations? The sex of the most recent partner? The sex of the majority of partners during one's lifetime? If the latter, at what point in an individual's lifetime can "majority of partners" be determined with accuracy, short of one's death?

The self-identification view asserts that individuals' sexual orientation is identifiable based on their beliefs about themselves; if someone believes, for instance, that he or she is heterosexual, then he or she is heterosexual. This view fails to consider instances in which an individual may experience attraction towards a member of the same sex, but not classify such feelings as homoerotic (Stein, 1999).

The dispositional view seemingly melds the basic tenets of the behavioral and self-identification perspectives. According to this view, an individual's sexual orientation is a function of both his or her sexual desires and fantasies about sexual relations with members of a specific sex and his or her choice of sexual partner under ideal conditions. This perspective allows for the possibility that an individual may have a sexual orientation before he or she actually ever has sexual relations. This perspective is not, however, without its difficulties, in that it may not be possible to know what an individual's choice of partner would be under circumstances that do not exist.

The Kinsey scale of sexual orientation has been termed a dispositional one because it simultaneously considers an individual's sexual behavior, sexual desires, and sexual fantasies in determining sexual orientation and also recognizes that these features may be discordant within the same individual (Stein, 1999). Kinsey and colleagues explained:

[T]he rating which an individual receives has a dual basis. It takes account of his overt sexual experience and/or his psychosexual reactions. In the majority of instances, the two aspects of the history parallel, but sometimes they are not in accord. In the latter case, the rating of an individual must be based upon an evaluation of the relative importance of the overt and the psychic in his history . . . The position of an individual on this scale is always based upon the relation of the heterosexual to the homosexual in his history, rather than upon the actual amount of overt experience or psychic reaction (Kinsey, Pomeroy, and Martin, 1948: 647).

Sexual orientation has traditionally been viewed as a binary phenomenon: heterosexual and homosexual (Stein, 1999). This construction of sexual orientation does not permit the existence, for instance, of bisexuality, and is unable to explain situational same-sex behaviors, such as male-male sex in prison for the purpose of self-protection or due to force.

In contrast, the bipolar construction views sexual orientation along a continuum, with exclusive heterosexuality at one end and exclusive homosexuality at the other (Kinsey, Pomeroy, and Martin, 1948). The Kinsey seven-point scale reflects this polarity with respect to sexual experience and desires:

0 = exclusively heterosexual, no homosexual
1 = predominately heterosexual, only incidental homosexual
2 = predominately heterosexual, but more than incidental homosexual
3 = equally heterosexual and homosexual
4 = predominately homosexual but more than incidental heterosexual
5 = predominately homosexual, but only incidental heterosexual
6 = exclusively homosexual with no heterosexual
X = no social-sexual contacts or reactions (Kinsey, Pomeroy, and Martin, 1948).

However, Kinsey's conceptualization of sexuality as a heterosexual-homosexual continuum has been challenged by a number of researchers. Stein (1999) has criticized this schema, noting that the classification of bisexuals as equally heterosexual and homosexual fails to consider the diversity that exists within bisexuality. For instance, individuals may be strongly attracted to individuals of both the same sex and the opposite sex, or they may be moderately attracted to individuals of both sexes, or they may be weakly attracted to individuals of both sexes.

Storms (1979, 1980, 1981) has argued that sexual orientation may be conceived of along two axes: one axis represents the degree of attraction to individuals of the same sex-gender and the second axis refers to the degree of attraction to those of a different sex-gender. Individuals are mapped on this grid without regard to their own physical sex, that is, without regard to whether they are male or female, but only with reference to the sameness or differentness of their partner's sex. Consequently, a male and a female may share the same position on the grid, despite the difference in their sex.

Stein (1999) has advocated a variation of this grid, which would utilize the y-axis to indicate the degree of attraction to women and the x-axis to represent the degree of attraction to men. The resulting grid would group together those who are attracted to men or women. He has further suggested the addition of a third axis to represent the degree of attraction to members of a third sex-gender and a fourth axis to depict the sexual object choice, such as heterosexual women, homosexual men, etc. Shively and De Cecco (1977) asserted that sexual orientation reflects two different continua, one of which represents the degree of heterosexuality and the other of homosexuality. In addition, sexual orientation is comprised of two different aspects, the physical preference and the affectional preference, each of which consists of heterosexual and homosexual continua. The Sell Scale of Sexual Orientation, developed by Gonsiorek, Sell, and Weinsrich (1995), assesses the frequency and strength of sexual interests, the frequency of sexual contacts, and self-identity in degrees of heterosexuality, homosexuality, and bisexuality. Klein (1978) characterized both heterosexuality and homosexuality as limited, whereas bisexuality was perceived of as tolerating ambiguity. (For a detailed discussion of measures of sexual orientation, see chapter 7.)

Divergent perspectives have been voiced in an attempt to understand bisexuality. Arguments have been made to the effect that bisexuality does not exist (Altshuler, 1984), while other scholars have asserted that the concept of bisexuality as it is commonly used represents a cultural construct (Paul, 2000). Indeed,

personal views about sexuality in the abstract reflect wider cultural understandings, and affect, in turn, the concrete constructions people place on their own feelings and experiences and thereby affect their behavior. So it is essential to accept cultural understandings of sexuality as crucial data, while at the same time rejecting the scientific validity of their underlying premise (Blumstein and Schwartz, 1977: 31).

The conflict theory of bisexuality posits that sexual orientation is a dichotomous construct consisting of heterosexuality and homosexuality in opposition (Zinik, 2000). According to this theory, a bisexual individual must therefore be (1) experiencing confusion or identity conflict, (2) in a transitional phase that is masking the individual's true sexual orientation, and (3) self-identifying as bisexual in order to consciously deny or subconsciously defend against his or her true (homosexual) orientation. Zinik (2000) has noted that this theory implicitly assumes that homosexuality must cancel out heterosexuality, that is, that they cannot co-exist in the same individual. Further, this perspective suggests that because no individual would choose homosexuality voluntarily given the tremendous social costs associated with this orientation, any homosexual behavior is indicative of a homosexual orientation.

In contrast, the flexibility theory views bisexuality as the integration of heterosexual and homosexual identities. Unlike the conflict theory, the flexibility theory does not view bisexuality as inherently problematic (Zinik, 2000).

Researchers have attempted to distinguish between various categories of bisexuality, often differentiating such groupings based upon the duration of bisexual activity, the nature of the bisexual relationship, and/or the context in which the bisexual behavior occurs. Klein (1978, 1993), for instance, delineated four types of bisexuality: transitional, historical, sequential, and concurrent. *Transitional bisexuality* refers to a phase that some individuals pass through in their evolution from heterosexuality to homosexuality. An *historical bisexual* is an individual who has had both male and female partners during his or her lifetime. *Sequential bisexuality* refers to individuals who have had relationships with both men and women, but with only one sex at a time, while *concurrent bisexuality* refers to individuals who have sexual relations with a male and a female partner during the same period of time. These and additional categorizations are set forth in Table 4, below.

The incidence of heterosexuality, homosexuality, and bisexuality is difficult to assess in view of the ambiguity and the complexity of these terms. As indicated previously, sexual orientation reflects a complex interaction between sexual attraction or desire, sexual behavior, and self-identification. Rodríguez Rust (2000: 292) has explained:

The fact that the terms *homosexual* and *heterosexual* can now refer to both individual sexual self-identities and to relationships involving people with such self-identities creates even more of a linguistic nightmare than has heretofore existed. Does heterosexual now refer to

TABLE 4. Classification systems of bisexuality

Study	Classification system: term and definition
Boulton (1991)	Bisexuality Adolescent bisexuality Married homosexual men Prostitution Situational homosexuality
Diamond (1998)	*Primary bisexuality*: individual is erotically aroused by both sexes regardless of sexual behavior *Secondary bisexuality*: individual engages in behavior with both sexes regardless of sexual arousal
Doll, Peterson, Magaña, and Carrier (1991)	Behavioral bisexual men Primary heterosexual relationships No primary heterosexual relationships Inaccessible heterosexual relationships
Klein (1978, 1993)	*Transitional*: phase that some individuals pass through in their evolution from heterosexuality to homosexuality *Historical*: individual who has had male and female partners during the course of his or her lifetime *Serial*: person who has had relationships with both males and females but not during the same time *Concurrent*: individual as had relationships with males and females during the same time period
McDonald (1982)	Transitory Transitional Enduring
Ross (1991)	*Defense bisexuality*: individual engages in bisexual behavior because culture in which he or she is situated discourages or condemns self-identification as gay/homosexual *Latin bisexuality*: refers to cultures in which insertive sex with a partner of either sex is considered to be consistent with heterosexual self-identity *Ritual bisexuality*: refers to bisexuality in cultures that accept same-sex behavior during certain phases of life without an association to homosexuality or bisexuality *Married:* refers to cultures in which individuals are obliged to marry and consequently maintain same-sex relations extramaritally *Experimental/Secondary*: individuals who are otherwise heterosexual engage in bisexual behavior *Equal:* individuals who are attracted to individuals of both sexes or who are attracted to people regardless of their sex *Technical*: refers to sexual relations in which a partner is not of the sex that they appear to be
Stokes and Miller (1998)	Behavioral bisexual men Men in transition Experimenters Opportunity-driven men Men with dual involvement
Weinberg, Williams, and Pryor (1994)	Classification system utilizes Kinsey scale to assess three dimensions: sexual feelings, sexual behaviors, and romantic feelings *Pure:* Kinsey 3 in all dimensions *Mid:* Kinsey 3 in one dimension and 2–4 in other two dimensions *Heterosexual-leaning*: Kinsey 2–4 in all dimensions *Homosexual-leaning*: Kinsey 4–6 in all dimensions *Varied:* Kinsey scores spread too widely to be encompassed by other formulated categories

the similarity or difference between one's own sex and the sex of one's preferred partners, to one's own sexual self-identity or essence, or to the relationship between two people each with their own sexual self-identities based on the sex of the people each is attracted to—which might bear no relation to the sex of the person they are currently involved with? (Emphasis in original.)

Indeed, research strongly indicates that sexual self-identity does not necessarily converge with sexual behavior or sexual attraction. As an example, the term "men who have sex with men" (MSM), defines neither bisexual men nor homosexual men, but includes them both, as well as men who may self-identify as heterosexual but who also have sexual relations with other men. The findings of several research studies, contained in Table 5, below, further support this premise. (For a full discussion of study findings related to the incidence and prevalence of various sexual orientations and the (non)convergence of the behavior with self-identity, see Rodríguez Rust, 2000).

In her review of the literature relating to various aspects of bisexuality, Rodríguez Rust (2000) observed that:

• Individuals can display homosexuality or heterosexuality in any one or more of three domains: sexual attraction, sexual behavior, and sexual identity
• The incidence of heterosexual, homosexual, or bisexual behavior, attraction, and/or identity depends on the point in time and length of the time period during which the behavior, attraction, or identity is being assessed.
• Responses regarding lifetime sexual experience vary depending on whether respondents are permitted to use their own definitions and terms to refer to their behavior or whether they are forced to choose from a preformulated listing.
• Sexual behavior, sexual attraction, and sexual identity are not necesarily congruent.
• Self-identity does not predict sexual behavior.

The lack of congruence between behavior and self-identity and Rust's observations necessarily raise the question as to why individuals self-define in noncongruent ways and why different studies suggest differing prevalences of various behaviors. Several explanations come to mind.

First, the formation of sexual identity is often a process, rather than an event. Scholars have conceived of it in a stage fashion, whereby an individual first becomes aware of his or her same-sex attraction, then begins to experiment, and ultimately accepts his or her same-sex orientation and discloses it publicly (Cass, 1979; Coleman, 1982; Troiden, 1989). Many of these models, however, fail to distinguish between the internal processes of awareness and decisionmaking and external processes involving the development of relationships, disclosure, and community involvement (Parks, Hughes, and Matthews, 2004). An individual's self-definition may vary depending on where he or she is in this process.

Second, the behaviors in question may be societally sanctioned, depending upon the time and place of the study. In such situations, individuals may be reticent to disclose accurately their self-identity and/or sexual behaviors. As an example,

TABLE 5. Selected studies indicating prevalence of sexual behavior in comparison with sexual identity

Study	Sample	Findings
Billy, Tanfer, Grady, and Keplinger (1993)	1991 National Survey of Men	Among respondents who had had same-sex contact during the previous 10 years: 57% of those aged 25–29 also had heterosexual contact during the same period 82% of those aged 30–34 also reported heterosexual contact
Carballo-Diéguez and Dolezal (1994)		Among Latino men who have sex with men (MSM) who had had at least one male partner during the previous year: 20% self-identified as bisexual or *hombres modernos* (modern men), 10% self-identified as heterosexual, 65% self-identified as gay, and 4% self-identified as drag queens 80% of those self-identifying as bisexual had had sex with a woman during the previous year, in comparison with 63% of the men self-identifying as heterosexual Almost three-fifths of the men self-identifying as gay had had sexual relations with a woman; 8% had had sex with a woman during the previous year
Cook et al. (1983)	65,471 men and 14,963 women responding to *Playboy* 133-item survey	8% of self-identified heterosexual men and women had had adult same-sex experiences Nearly 20% of women had had adolescent same-sex sexual experiences 35% of all male respondents regardless of sexual orientation had ever had homosexual experiences
Harry (1990)	American Broadcasting Company-*Washington Post* 1985 telephone poll in all 50 states, using national probability sample to assess attitudes regarding social and political issues	Of 633 male respondents, 3.7% found to be homosexual or bisexual in attraction
Hunt (1974)	2,026 individuals sampled through random selection of homes in 24 U.S. cities	7% of men and 11% of women masturbated to same-sex fantasies 17–18% of men reported homosexual experiences after the onset of adolescence 1% of men and 0.5% of women self-identified as mainly or totally homosexual 9% of married women and 12–13% of married men had at least 1 same-sex experience

(Continued)

TABLE 3. (Continued)

Study	Sample	Findings
Laumann, Gagnon, Michael, and Michaels (1994)	National Health and Social Life Survey (NHSLS): multistage area probability sampling of English-speaking U.S. residents aged 18–59; 17% of those selected refused participation; final sample included 3,432 men and women	4.3% of women and 9.1% of men engaged in some same-sex activity since puberty 4.1% of women and 4.9% of men had engaged in same-sex behavior since the age of 18 1.3% of sexually active women and 2.7% of sexually active men had engaged in same-sex behavior during the previous year Among those who had had same sex partners, 90.7% of women and 94.9% of men had had partners of both sexes since puberty Among those who had had same sex partners, 62.9% of women and 51.6% of men had partners of both sexes in the past 5 years Among those who had had same sex partners, 25.0% of women and 25.3% of men had had partners of both sexes in the previous year 5.8% of all men and 3.3% of all women had had both male and female partners since puberty BUT 0.5% of women and 0.8% of men self-identified as bisexual 0.6% of men and 0.2% of women indicated that they had had sex exclusively with same-sex partners since puberty BUT 0.9% of women and 2.0% of men self-identified as homosexual, gay, or lesbian
Sell, Wells, and Wypij (1995)	Center for Health Affairs Survey	3.6% of women and 6.2% of men had same sex contact during previous 5 years 6.7% of women and 12.1% of men had same sex contact since the age of 15
Smith (1991)	1988 and 1989 General Social Survey	since age 18: 3% of adults have not been sexually active 91% of adults have been exclusively heterosexual 5.6% of adults have been bisexual 0.7% of adults have been exclusively homosexual

same-sex relations were, until relatively recently, punishable by imprisonment in various jurisdictions within the United States (*Lawrence v. Texas*, 2003) and continue to be punishable, sometimes by death, in other countries (International Lesbian and Gay Association, 1999). Even in the absence of legal prohibitions, individuals identifying as non-heterosexuals or admitting to non-heterosexual behaviors may face stigmatization and loss of opportunities, such as employment. This may be particularly true for bisexuals, who may be regarded as homosexuals by heterosexuals and resented for "passing" as heterosexuals by homosexuals. (This situation is reminiscent of the one drop rule, discussed in chapter 2, under which any drop of black blood was sufficient to justify classifying an individual as black. In the context of sexual behavior, any non-heterosexual liaison is deemed sufficient to justify classification of an individual by heterosexuals as homosexual, while any heterosexual behavior justifies for homosexuals the classification of an individual as heterosexual, or "passing.")

A review of past sexual research suggests that such concerns, to the extent that they exist, may not be misplaced. Unfortunately, sexual orientation research has often attempted to explain the basis of homosexuality, rather than focusing on an understanding of the origin of sexual orientation, regardless of the specific orientation. In contrast to same-sex behavior, but often with reference to heterosexuality as the standard, homosexuality has been conceived of as an innate, relatively stable condition (Murray, 1987); a congenital, but not hereditary, condition (Heller, 1981); a form of congenital degeneracy (Gindorf, 1977); an earlier, evolutionary form of the human race, that is, bisexual or hermaphroditic (Krafft-Ebing, 1965); a perverse and immature orientation resulting from family interactions during childhood development (Dynes, 1987; Freud, 1920); and the result of psychological processes similar to those that lead to heterosexuality, modifiable through various forms of therapy (Akers, 1977). Prior to 1973, the American Psychiatric Association classified homosexuality as a form of mental illness (Greenberg, 1988). Clearly, in view of "the different positions of power that lesbians and gay men, as opposed to heterosexuals, have in most cultures, there exists an asymmetry in how the origins of sexual orientation are explored and a recurring pattern of who asks such questions and in what contexts these questions are asked" (Stein, 1999: 331).

Many of the studies that gave rise to these conclusions are characterized by serious methodological flaws, including selection bias, due to a reliance on convenience samples; misclassification, due to inaccurate mechanisms for the assessment of sexual orientation; and inadequate statistical power due to a relatively small sample size (Stein, 1999). In addition, correlations that are noted are often misinterpreted as being indicative of a causal relationship when, in fact, no such inference can be made due to the cross-sectional nature of the particular study. The dissemination of these study findings in the absence of a more complete understanding of human sexuality on the part of the researchers and/or their reading audience may have further perpetuated negative attitudes towards non-heterosexuality and non-heterosexuals. This may be particularly problematic for individuals claiming a bisexual identity, who are often viewed simultaneously as homosexual within heterosexual communities and as "double agents" within homosexual and lesbian communities, suffering stigmatization from both (Hemmings, 1993; Ochs, 1996).

Third, the manner in which the questions are phrased may have significant impact on the responses. An inappropriate word choice by the investigator may lead to under- or overestimates of a behavior or perspective, from which conclusions are then drawn. As seen in the study conducted by Carballo-Diéguez and Dolezal (1994), above, insight into individuals' sexual activities and identities may be heightened when they are permitted to self-label rather than being asked to select their response from a listing that has been preformulated by the investigator. Additionally, responses may differ depending upon the time frame for the behavior in question (for example, lifetime, last five years, previous year), the focus of the question (sexual orientation, sexual identity, sexual attraction, or sexual activities), and the format of the question (for instance, a scale versus a simple, yes/no response).

Definitional issues may also be critical in the formulation of the questions. As an example, a question that is framed in terms of "sexual contact" may be interpreted by respondents to refer to any sexual contact, including kissing, or to only relations involving genital contact. The word "intercourse" is similarly ambiguous, as it can refer to vaginal intercourse, anal intercourse, and oral intercourse. It is also unclear whether this term encompasses the use of sex toys, such as dildos and vibrators, for penetrative sex. The use of the word "gay," for instance, may convey a significantly different meaning than the word "homosexual" which, as discussed earlier, differs in meaning from the term "men who have sex with men." Individuals may self-identify as gay and/or as homosexual and/or as a man who has sex with men:

Homosexual was the label that was applied to Gay people as a device for separating us from the rest of the population .... Gay is a descriptive label we have assigned to ourselves as a way of reminding ourselves and others that awareness of our sexuality facilitates a capability rather than creating a restriction. It means that we are capable of fully loving a person of the same gender .... But the label does not limit us (Clark, 1977: 103–106).

The term "gay," unlike the term "homosexual," evolved through the Gay Liberation Movement to embody political connotations. Gays were redefined as a stigmatized minority, and the concept of the gay community emerged (Paul, 2000). Accordingly, the choice of the term to be used may differ depend upon the information sought and may be critical to respondents' understanding of the question.

Finally, the manner in which the sample of individuals participating in the study is constructed may affect the study findings. Convenience samples drawn from particular locales, such as bars, bathhouses, prisons, social service organizations, etc. may not include individuals who would be reached through other techniques, such as random digit dialing and may, consequently, reflect biases in the selection of participants, thereby limiting the generalizability of the findings to other populations or the population as a whole.

Summary

Although sex, gender, and sexual orientation are often perceived as simple concepts, it is clear from this review that they are quite complex. This chapter has underscored the importance of clarity in formulating the research question, in identifying the reference group of interest, and in specifying the meaning of the terms that are used in research. The lack of clarity often impedes a comparison of findings across studies, even in regard to the same populations.

References

Akers, R.L. (1977). *Deviant Behavior: A Social Learning Approach*. Belmont, California: Wadsworth.

Altshuler, K.Z. (1984). On the question of bisexuality. *American Journal of Psychotherapy* 38(4): 484–493.

Ames, J. (Ed.). (2005). *Sexual Metamorphoses: An Anthology of Transsexual Memoirs*. New York: Vintage Books.

Badinter, E. (1995). *XY: On Masculine Identity*. (Trans. L. Davis). New York: Columbia University Press.

Bakker, A., van Kesteren, F.J.M., Gooren, L.J.G., Bezemer, P.D. (1993). The prevalence of transsexualism in the Netherlands. *Acta Psychiatrica Scandinavia* 87: 237–238.

Barrett, W.P. (Trans.). (1931). *The Trial of Jeanne d"Arc*. London: Routledge.

Bartky, S. (1990). *Femininity and Domination: Studies in the Phenomenology of Oppression*. New York: Routledge.

Billy, J.O.G., Tanfer, K., Grady, W.R., Klepinger, D.H. (1993). The sexual behavior of men in the United States. *Family Planning Perspectives* 25: 52–60.

Blumstein, P.W., Schwartz, P. (1977). Bisexuality: Some social-psychological issues. *Journal of Social Issues* 33: 30–45.

Bolin, A. (1992). Coming of age among transsexuals. In T.L. Whitehead, B.V. Reid (Eds.), *Gender Constructs and Social Issues* (pp. 13–39). Chicago: University of Chicago Press.

Boulton, M. (1991). Review of the literature on bisexuality and HIV transmission. In R.A.P. Tielman, M. Carballo, A.C. Hendriks (Eds.), *Bisexuality and HIV/AIDS: A Global Perspective* (pp. 187–209). Buffalo, New York: Prometheus.

Brannon, R. (1976). The male sex role—and what it's done for us lately. In R. Brannon, D. David (Eds.), *The Forty-Nine Percent Majority: The Male Sex Role* (pp. 1–40). Boston: Addison-Wesley.

Brevard, A. (2001). *The Woman I Was Not Born to Be: A Transsexual Journey*. Philadelphia, Pennsylvania: Temple University Press.

Brierley, H. (2000). Gender identity and sexual behaviour. In P.C. Rodríguez Rust (Ed.), *Bisexuality in the United States* (pp. 104–126). New York: Columbia University Press.

Butler, J. (1985). Embodied identity in De Beauvoir's *The Second Sex*. Unpublished manuscript, presented to American Philosophical Association, March 22. Quoted in S.L. Bartky. (1990). *Femininity and Domination: Studies in the Phenomenology of Oppression*. New York: Routledge.

Carballo-Diéguez, A., Dolezal, C. (1994). Contrasting types of Puerto Rican men who have sex with men (MSM). *Journal of Psychology and Human Sexuality* 6(4): 41–67.

Cass, V. (1979). Homosexual identity formation: A theoretical model. *Journal of Homosexuality* 4(3): 219–235.

Chodorow, N. (1978). *The Reproduction of Mothering*. Berkeley, California: University of California Press.

Coleman, E. (1982). Developmental stages in the coming-out process. In W. Paul, J.D. Weinrich, J.C. Gonsiorek, M.E. Hotvedt (Eds.), *Homosexuality: Social, Psychological, and Biological Issues* (pp. 144–158). Beverly Hills, California: Sage.

Connell, R.W. (2005). *Masculinities*, 2nd ed. Berkeley, California: University of California Press.

Cook, K., in collaboration with Kretchner, A., Nellis, B., Lever, J., Hertz, R. (1983). The Playboy readers' sex survey: Part three. *Playboy* (May): 126, 128, 136, 210–212, 215–216, 219–220.

Crichton, D. (1992). Gender reassignment surgery for male primary transsexuals. *South African Medical Journal* 83: 347–349.

Deutsch, H. (1944). *The Psychology of Women*, vol. 1. New York: Grune & Stratton.

Deutsch, H. (1944). *The Psychology of Women*, vol. 2. New York: Grune & Stratton.

Diamond, M. (1998). Bisexuality: A biological perspective. In E.J. Haeberle, R. Gindorf (Eds.), *Bisexualities: The Ideology and Practice of Sexual Contact with Both Men and Women* (pp. 53–80). New York: Continuum.

Doll, L.S., Peterson, L.R., Magaña, J.R., Carrier, J.M. (1991). Male bisexuality and AIDS in the United States. In R. Tielman, M. Carballo, A. Hendriks (Eds.), *Bisexuality and HIV/AIDS: A Global Perspective* (pp. 27–39). Buffalo, New York: Prometheus.

Doyle, J.A. (1989). *The Male Experience*, 2nd ed. Dubuque, Iowa: William C. Brown.

Dreger, A.D. (1998). *Hermaphrodites and the Medical Invention of Sex*. Cambridge, Massachusetts: Harvard University Press.

Duvall, E.M., Hill, R. (1947). *When You Marry*. New York: Association Press.

Dynes, W. (1987). *Homosexuality: A Research Guide*. New York: Garland.

Easthope, A. (1986). *What a Man's Gotta Do: The Masculine Myth in Popular Culture*. London: Paladin/Grafton.

Eldh, J. (1993). Construction of a neovagina with preservation of the glans penis as a clitoris in male transsexuals. *Plastic Reconstructive Surgery* 91: 895–900.

Ellis, H. (1908). *Studies in the Psychology of Sex: Sexual Inversion*, 2nd ed. Philadelphia: F.A. Davis Co. Cited in A.D. Dreger. (1998). *Hermaphrodites and the Medical Invention of Sex*. Cambridge, Massachusetts: Harvard University Press.

Feinberg, L. (1996). *Transgender Warriors*. Boston: Beacon Press.

Freud, S. (1961). Femininity, new introductory lectures. In J. Strachey (Ed.). *Standard Edition of the Complete Psychological Works of Sigmund Freud*, vol. 19. London: Hogarth Press.

Freud, S. (1920). The psychogenesis of a case of homosexuality in a woman. In P. Rieff (Ed.). (1963). *Sexuality and the Psychology of Love* (pp. 133–159). New York: Collier.

Friedan, B. (1963). *The Feminine Mystique*. New York: W.W. Norton & Company.

Garber, M. (1992). *Vested Interests: Cross-Dressing and Cultural Anxiety*. New York: HarperCollins.

Gaylin, W. (1992). *The Male Ego*. New York: Viking.

Gilligan, J. (2001). *Preventing Violence*. New York: Thames & Hudson.

Gindorf, R. (1977). Wissenschaftliche Ideologien im Wandel: Die Angst von der Homosexualitat als intellektuelles Ereignis. In J.S. Hohmann (Ed.). *Der underdruckte Sexus* (pp. 129–144). Berlin: Andreas Achenbach Lollar. Cited in D.F. Greenberg. (1988). *The Construction of Homosexuality*. Chicago: University of Chicago Press.

Godlewski, J. (1988). Transsexualism and anatomic sex: Ratio reversal in Poland. *Archives of Sexual Behavior* 17: 547–548.

Gonsiorek, J.C., Sell, R.L., Weinrich, J.D. (1995). Definition and measurement of sexual orientation. *Suicide and Life-Threatening Behavior* 25 (Supplement): 40–51.

Gordon, E.B. (1991). Transsexual healing: Medicaid funding of sex reassignment surgery. *Archives of Sexual Behavior* 20: 61–79.

Greenberg, D.F. (1988). *The Construction of Homosexuality*. Chicago: University of Chicago Press.

Griggs, C. (2004). *Journal of a Sex Change: Passage through Trinidad*. Oxford, U.K.: Berg.

Groveman, S.A. (1999). The Hanukkah bush: Ethical implications in the clinical management of intersex. In A.D. Dreger (Ed.). *Intersex in the Age of Ethics* (pp. 23–28). Hagerstown, Maryland: University Publishing Group, Inc.

Hage, J.J., Bloem, J.J.A.M., Suliman, H.M. (1993). Review of the literature on techniques for phalloplasty with emphasis on the applicability in female-to-male transsexuals. *Journal of Urology* 150: 1093–1098.

Hage, J.J., Bouman, F.G., de Graaf, F.H., Bloem, J.J.A.M. (1993). Construction of the neophallus in female-to-male transsexuals: The Amsterdam experience. *Journal of Urology* 149: 1463–1468.

Hage, J.J., Bout, C.A., Bloem, J.J.A.M., Megens, J.A.J. (1993). Phalloplasty in female-to-male transsexuals: What do our patients ask for? *Annals of Plastic Surgery* 30: 323–326.

Harry, J. (1990). A probability sample of gay males. *Journal of Homosexuality* 19 (1): 89–104.

Havemann, E., West, P.S. (1952). *They Went to College: The College Graduate in America Today.* New York: Harcourt, Brace & Company.

Heller, P. (1981). A quarrel over bisexuality. In G. Chapple, H.H. Schulte (Eds.). *The Turn of the Century: German Literature and Art, 1890–1915* (pp. 87–115). Bonn: Bouvier Verlag Herbert Grundmann.

Hemmings, C. (1993). Resituating the bisexual body: From identity to difference. In J. Bristow, A.R. Wilson (Eds.), *Activating Theory: Lesbian, Gay, & Bisexual Politics* (pp. 118–138). London: Lawrence and Wishart.

Heriot, A. (1975). *The Castrati in Opera.* New York: Da Capo Press.

Humphreys, L. (1970). *Tearoom Trade: Impersonal Sex in Public Places.* Chicago: Aldine.

Hunt, M. (1974). *Sexual Behavior in the 1970s.* Chicago: Playboy.

International Lesbian and Gay Association. (1999). World Legal Survey. Available at http://www.ilga.info/Information/Legal_survey/Summary%20information/death_penalty_for_homosexual_act.htm. Last accessed September 21, 2005.

Jagiello, G., Atwell, J.D. (1962). Prevalence of testicular feminisation. *Lancet* ii: 329.

Josso, N. (1981). Physiology of sex differentiation: A guide to understanding and management of the intersex child. In N. Josso (Ed.). *Pediatric and Adolescent Endocrinology, vol. 8: The Intersex Child* (pp. 1–13). Basel, Switzerland: S. Karger.

Just Evelyn. (1998). *"...Mom, I Need to Be a Girl."* Imperial Beach, California: Walter Trook Publishing.

Kessler, S.J. (1998). *Lessons from the Intersexed.* New Brunswick, New Jersey: Rutgers University Press.

Kimmel, M.S. (2003). Masculinity as homophobia. In E. Disch (Ed.). *Reconstructing Gender: A Multicultural Anthology.* Boston: McGraw Hill.

Kinsey, A., Pomeroy, W., Martin, C. (1948). *Sexual Behavior in the Human Male.* Philadelphia: W.B. Saunders.

Kismaric, C., Heiferman, M. (1996). *Growing Up with Dick and Jane: Learning and Living the American Dream.* New York: HarperCollins.

Klein, F. (1993). *The Bisexual Option*, 2nd ed. New York: Harrington Park.

Klein, F. (1978). *The Bisexual Option: A Concept of One-Hundred Percent Intimacy.* New York: Arbor House.

Komisar, L. (1976). Violence and the masculine mystique. In D.S. David, R. Brannon (Eds.). *The Forty-Nine Percent Majority: The Male Sex Role.* Boston: Addison-Wesley.

Krafft-Ebing, R.V. (1965). *Psychopathia Sexualis: A Medico-Forensic Study* (H.E. Wedeck, Trans.). New York: G.P. Putnam's Sons [original work pub. 1886].

Krob, G., Braun, A., Kuhnle, U. (1994). Hermaphroditism: Geographical distribution, clinical findings, chromosomes and gonadal histology. *European Journal of Pediatrics* 153: 2–10.

Laumann, E.O., Gagnon, J.H., Michael, R.T., Michaels, S. (1994). *The Social Organization of Sexuality: Sexual Practices in the United States.* Chicago: University of Chicago Press.

Lawrence v. Texas. (2003). 539 U.S. 558.

Levant, R.F. (1995). Toward the reconstruction of masculinity. In R.F. Levant, W.S. Pollack (Eds.). *A New Psychology of Men* (pp. 229–251). New York: Basic Books.

Leverenz, D. (1986). Manhood, humiliation, and public life: Some stories. *Southwest Review,* 71.

Lillie, F. (1939). General biological introduction. In E. Allen (Ed.), *Sex and Internal Secretions: A Survey of Recent Research,* 2nd ed. Baltimore, Maryland: Williams and Wilkins.

Ludden, A. (1956). *Plain Talk for Women Under 21!* New York: Dodd, Mead, and Company.

Martin, D. (1964). *Taffy's Tips to Teens.* Englewood Cliffs, New Jersey: Prentice-Hall, Inc.

Martin, M. (1977). *Emergence: A Transsexual Autobiography.* New York: Crown Publishers, Inc.

McDonald, A.P., Jr. (1982). Research on sexual orientation: A bridge that touches both shores but doesn't meet in the middle. *Journal of Sex Education and Therapy* 8: 9–13. [Cited by Rodríguez Rust, 2000].

Messner, M.A. (2003). Boyhood, organized sports, and the construction of masculinities. In E. Disch (Ed.). *Reconstructing Gender: A Multicultural Anthology* (pp. 110–126). Boston: McGraw Hill.

Mignon, C.J., Brown, T.R., Fichman, K.R. (1981). Androgen insensitivity syndrome. In N. Josso (Ed.). *Pediatric and Adolescent Endocrinology, vol. 8: The Intersex Child* (pp. 171–202). Basel, Switzerland: S. Karger.

Molloy, J.T. (1977). *The Woman's Dress for Success Book.* New York: Warner Books.

Money, J., Erhardt, A. (1972). *Man and Woman, Boy and Girl.* Baltimore, Maryland: Johns Hopkins University Press.

Moore, K.L. (1989). *Before We Are Born: Basic Embryology and Birth Defects,* 3rd ed. Philadelphia: W.B. Saunders Company.

Moore, K.L., Persaud, T.V.N. (1993). *The Developing Human: Clinically Oriented Embryology* (5th ed.). Philadelphia, Pennsylvania: W.B. Saunders.

Murray, S.O. (1987). Homosexual acts and selves in early modern Europe. *Journal of Homosexuality* 15: 421–439.

Nanda, S. (1994). Hijras: An alternative sex and gender role in India. In G. Herdt (Ed.), *Third Sex, Third Gender: Beyond Sexual Dimorphism in Culture and History* (pp. 373–417). New York: Zone Books.

Nanda, S. (1990). *Neither Man Nor Woman: The Hijras of India.* Belmont, California: Wadsworth Publishing Company.

Noble, V. (1992). A helping hand from the guys. In K.L. Hagan (Ed.). *Women Respond to the Men's Movement.* San Francisco, California: HarperCollins.

Notman, M. (1982). Feminine development: Changes in psychoanalytic theory. In C.C. Nadelson, M.T. Notman (Eds.). *The Woman Patient, vol. 2: Concepts of Femininity and the Life Cycle* (pp. 3–29). New York: Plenum Press.

Ochs, R. (1996). Biphobia: It goes more than two ways. In B.A. Firestein (Ed.), Bisexuality: *The Psychology of an Invisible Minority* (pp. 217–239). Thousand Oaks, California: Sage.

O'Neil, J.M. (1982). Gender-role conflict and strain in men's lives. In K. Solomon, N. Levy (Eds.). *Men in Transition: Theory and Therapy* (pp. 5–44). New York: Plenum.

Parks, C.A., Hughes, T.L., Matthews, A.K. (2004). Race/ethnicity and sexual orientation: Intersecting identities. *Cultural Diversity and Ethnic Minority Psychology* 10(3): 241–254.

Paul, J.P. (2000). Bisexuality: Reassessing our paradigms of sexuality. In P.C. Rodríguez Rust (Ed.), *Bisexuality in the United States* (pp. 11–23). New York: Columbia University Press.

Pauley, I.B. (1968). The current status of the change of sex operation. *Journal of Nervous and Mental Disease* 147: 460–471.

Reid, W.H., Wise, M.G. (1995). *DSM-IV Training Guide*. New York: Brunner Mazel.

Robinson, L.W. (1960). How to know when you're really feminine. *Good Housekeeping, June,* 2.

Rodríguez Rust, P.C. (2000). Alternatives to binary sexuality: Modeling bisexuality. In P.C. Rodríguez Rust (Ed.), *Bisexuality in the United States* (pp. 33–54). New York: Columbia University Press.

Roscoe, W. (1994). How to become a berdache: Toward a unified theory of gender diversity. In G. Herdt (Ed.), *Third Sex, Third Gender: Beyond Sexual Dimorphism in Culture and History* (pp. 329–372). New York: Zone Books.

Roscoe, W. (1991). *The Zuni Man-Woman.* Albuquerque, New Mexico: University of New Mexico Press.

Rodríguez Rust, P.C. (2000). Review of statistical findings. In P.C. Rodríguez Rust (Ed.), *Bisexuality in the United States* (pp. 129–184). New York: Columbia University Press.

Ross, M. (1991). A taxonomy of global behavior. In R. Tielman, M. Carballo, A. Hendriks (Eds.), *Bisexuality and HIV/AIDS: A Global Perspective* (p. 21–26). Buffalo, New York: Prometheus.

Rothblatt, M. (1995). *The Apartheid of Sex: A Manifesto in the Freedom of Gender.* New York: Crown Publishers.

Sapino, A., Pietribiasi, F., Godano, A., Bussolati, G. (1992). Effect of long-term administration of androgens on breast tissues of female-to-male transsexuals. *Annals of the New York Academy of Science* 586: 143–145.

Scott-Maxwell, F. (1958). Should mothers of young children work? *Ladies' Home Journal, November,* 156, 158.

Sell, R.L., Wells, J.A., Wypij, D. (1995). The prevalence of homosexual behavior and attraction in the United States, the United Kingdom, and France: Results of national population-based samples. *Archives of Sexual Behavior* 24(3): 235–248.

Shively, M.G., De Cecco, J.P. (1977). Components of sexual identity. *Journal of Homosexuality* 3(1): 41–48.

Smith, T.W. (1991). Adult sexual behavior in 1989: Number of partners, frequency of intercourse and risk of AIDS. *Family Planning Perspectives* 23(3): 102–107.

Stein, E. (1999). *The Mismeasure of Desire: The Science, Theory, and Ethics of Sexual Orientation.* Oxford, U.K.: Oxford University Press.

Stein, M., Tiefer, L., Melman, A. (1990). Followup observations of operated male-to-female transsexuals. *Journal of Urology* 143: 1188–1192.

Stepan, N.L. (1990). Race and gender: The role of analogy in science. In D.T. Goldberg (Ed.), *Anatomy of Racism* (pp. 38–57). Minneapolis, Minnesota: University of Minnesota Press.

Stokes, J.P., Miller, R.L. (1998). Toward an understanding of behaviourally bisexual men: The influence of context and culture. *Canadian Journal of Human Sexuality* 7(2): 101–113.

Stoller, R.J. (1968). *Sex and Gender: On the Development of Masculinity and Femininity.* New York: Science House.

Storms, M. (1979). Sex-role identity and its relationship to sex-role attributes and sex-role stereotypes. *Journal of Personality and Social Psychology* 37: 1779–1789.

Storms, M. (1980). Theories of sexual orientation. *Journal of Personality and Social Psychology* 38: 783–792.

Storms, M. (1981). A theory of erotic orientation development. *Psychological Review* 88: 340–353.

Stouffer, S.A., Lumsdaine, A.A., Lumsdaine, M.H., Williams, R.M., Jr., Smith, M.B., Janis, I.L., Star, S.A., Cottrell, L.S. (1976). Masculinity and the role of the combat soldier. In R. Brannon, D. David (Eds.), *The Forty-Nine Percent Majority: The Male Sex Role*. Boston: Addison-Wesley.

Talerman, A., Verp, M.S., Senekjian, E., Gilewski, T., Vogelzang, N. (1990). True hermaphrodite with bilateral ovotestes, bilateral gonadoblastomas and the dysgerminomas, 46,XX/46,XY karotype, and a successful pregnancy. *Cancer* 66: 2668–2671.

Thompson, M.W., McInnes, R.R., Willard, H.F. (1991). *Thompson & Thompson Genetics in Medicine*, 5th ed. Philadelphia: W.B. Saunders & Company.

Trexler, R.C. (1995). *Sex and Conquest: Gendered Violence, Political Order, and the European Conquest of the Americas*. Ithaca, New York: Cornell University Press.

Troiden, R.R. (1989). The formation of homosexual identities. *Journal of Homosexuality* 17(1/2): 43–73.

Valenta, L.J., Elias, A.N., Domurat, E.S. (1992). Hormone pattern in pharmacologically feminized male transsexuals in the California state prison system. *Journal of the American Medical Association* 84: 241–250.

Vance, C.S. (1995). Social construction theory and sexuality. In M. Berger, B. Wallis, S. Watson (Eds.). *Constructing Masculinity* (pp. 37–48). New York: Routledge.

Walinder, J. (1967). *Transsexualism: A Study of Forty-Three Cases* (H. Fry, Trans.). Stockholm: Scandinavian University Books.

Weinberg, M.S., Williams, C.J., Pryor, D.W. (1994). *Dual Attraction: Understanding Bisexuality*. New York: Oxford University Press.

Whitehead, S.M., Barrett, F.J. (2001). The sociology of masculinity. In S.M. Whitehead, F.J. Barrett (Eds.), *The Masculinities Reader* (pp. 1–26). Malden, Massachusetts: Blackwell Publishers Inc.

Williams, W.L. (1992). *The Spirit and the Flesh: Sexual Diversity in American Indian Culture*. Boston: Beacon Press.

Wilson, B.E., Reiner, W.G. (1999). Management of intersex: A shifting paradigm. In A.D. Dreger (Ed.). *Intersex in the Age of Ethics* (pp. 119–135). Hagerstown, Maryland: University Publishing Group, Inc.

Wilson, J.D. (1992). Syndromes of androgen resistance. *Biology of Reproduction* 46: 168–173.

Woolfolk R.I., Richardson, F. (1978). *Sanity, Stress, and Survival*. New York: Signet.

Young, A. (2000). *Women Who Become Men: Albanian Sworn Virgins*. Oxford, U.K.: Berg.

Zinik, G. (2000). Identity conflict or adaptive flexibility? Bisexuality reconsidered. In P.C. Rodríguez Rust (Ed.), *Bisexuality in the United States* (pp. 55–60). New York: Columbia University Press.

5
Race, Ethnicity, and Sexual Orientation in Health

Ethnicity, Race, and Related Constructs in Health Research

Despite the lack of consensus regarding the precise definitions and categories of ethnicity, race, sexual orientation and related constructs, researchers continue to utilize them in health-related research, often without adequate explanation of their meaning and/or significance within a particular context. This chapter reviews recent research findings that have focused on race, ethnicity, and sexual orientation on the one hand, and health, health care, and/or health care utilization on the other. The strengths and weaknesses of the various approaches used to operationalize these constructs in the research are explored, recognizing, however, that perfect studies do not exist. This discussion is intended to provoke thought as to how we might better define these constructs in the context of research to facilitate the application of research findings to a practice setting and to enhance comparability in the use of these constructs across studies. It is not possible, however, to provide a comprehensive examination of all such research within the scope of a single chapter, and readers are advised to consult with other resources for further discussion in a particular area.

Health Care Services

The careful delineation of concepts of race and ethnicity may be critical to understand patterns of health and health care seeking and utilization, as well as variations in the quality of and satisfaction with health care across various groups. Depending upon the focus of a particular investigation, race/ethnicity as perceived by the relevant observer(s) may actually be more informative than self-identified race/ethnicity. For instance, individuals may receive differential treatment from providers when provider race/ethnicity is different from their own (Krieger, Sidney, and Coakley, 1998) or may face financial and language barriers to access even though fully insured (Karter, Ferrara, Darbinian, Ackerman, and Selby, 2000).

Past research suggests that access varies across racial/ethnic groups. An investigation involving 3,689 individuals over the age of 65 living in a 108-county area in western Texas found that being Hispanic predicted not having a usual source of care (Rohrer, Kruse, and Zhang, 2004). Unfortunately, "ethnicity" was categorized as "Non-Hispanic white, Hispanic, or of other races," and the investigators did not specify how race/ethnicity was determined. The authors concluded that additional outreach was necessary to increase the opportunity for individuals to have a regular source of care. However, various other barriers may have existed, including language, discrimination, and income. Language discordance between a provider and patient, for instance, has been shown to constitute an important barrier to physician-patient agreement (Clark, Sleath, and Rubin, 2003). The opportunity to better understand the effect, if any, of these variables was lost because race and ethnicity were collapsed and data were not collected regarding language issues.

Another study that investigated participation by noninstitutionalized civilian individuals in health care settings across racial and ethnic groups during a 2-1/2 year period found that, as compared with whites, fewer blacks and Hispanics received care in physicians' office, outpatient clinics, and emergency departments, even after adjusting for potential confounders (Bliss, Meyers, Phillips, Jr., Fryer, Dovey, and Green, 2004). The researchers hypothesized that the lower rates of utilization of physicians' offices and outpatient clinics were potentially attributable to mistrust and perceived discrimination because of their racial or ethnic background. Because the analyses relied on a pre-existing national database, this possible explanation could not be explored further.

Other studies, however, suggest that this may be a plausible explanation for these findings. A study involving 537 primary care patients at a medical office indicated that patient satisfaction with the direct physician encounter was significantly less among nonwhite patients as compared to non-Hispanic white patients, even within a relatively affluent and well-educated patient population (Barr, 2004). Another investigation of patient-physician communication during medical visits that relied on questionnaires and audiotapes from 458 patients who visited 61 physicians over a four-year period found that physicians were 23% more verbally dominant and engaged in 33% less patient-centered communication with African American patients compared with white patients (Johnson, Roter, Powe, and Cooper, 2004). Research conducted by Weech-Maldonado and colleagues (2003) utilized data from the National CAHPS Benchmarking Database to examine whether reports and ratings of care by 49,327 adults enrolled in Medicaid managed care plans in 14 states varied by race/ethnicity and/or language. Unlike many other studies, this investigation utilized nine different racial/ethnic categories and further classified Hispanics, Asians, and whites based upon the language spoken at home. The researchers found that racial and ethnic minorities, and particularly individuals with limited English proficiency, reported worse care than English-speaking white patients. Such findings suggest that expectations of the physician encounter may vary across communities and/or that physicians and other healthcare providers may treat nonwhite patients differently than non-Hispanic white patients, regardless of their socioeconomic and educational levels (Barr, 2004; Weech-Maldonado, Morales, Elliott, Spritzer, Marshall, and Hays, 2003).

Various studies suggest that the quality of available health care varies across minority groups. An investigation of men's health care based on data obtained from several national databases indicated that compared to non-Hispanic whites, Hispanic men were significantly less likely to receive colorectal cancer screening, cardiovascular risk factor screening and management, and vaccinations, while black and Asian men were significantly less likely to receive adult immunizations and colorectal cancer screening (Feliz-Aaron, Moy, Kang, Patel, Chesley, and Clancy, 2005). Black men were also found to have received worse care for end-stage renal disease, and Hispanic and black men received lesser quality mental health services. Because the databases did not include information on numerous relevant factors, such as health status, comorbidities, and severity of illness, these represented unadjusted findings and it was not possible to identify the specific reason(s) for these disparities. Consequently, it is more difficult to evaluate the underlying meaning of the racial/ethnic differences that were reported.

Investigations of the quality of care in other settings have yielded similar conclusions. A study of emergency department wait times for 20,633 patient visits found that even after adjustment for hospital location, geographic region, and payer status, non-Hispanic black and Hispanic white patients waited longer than non-Hispanic white patients (James, Bourgeois, and Shannon, 2005). It could not be determined from the data whether this differential was attributable to discrimination, cultural incompetence, language barriers, or other factors.

Maternal and Child Health

Pregnancy and Delivery

Various research groups have concluded that coverage of information with recommended health promotion content is less adequate for African American women than it is for non-Hispanic white women. Kogan and colleagues (1994) reported that African American women were significantly less likely than Caucasian women to report receiving information on smoking and alcohol cessation during pregnancy, even after controlling for sociodemographic status, medical factors, and utilization of care. An earlier study had similarly found that African American women reported receiving less advice about alcohol use and more advice about cigarette use and the use of street drugs as compared with Caucasian women (Hiatt, Chin, and Croughan-Minihane, 1991). A cross-sectional study conducted by Vonderheid, Montgomery, and Norr (2003) examined the topics covered in prenatal care compared to the information that the study participants reported they needed. The study focused on self-identified English-speaking Mexican American and African American women; the study did not report length of residence in the U.S., place of birth, or immigration status, which potentially could have been implicated. The researchers found that the African American women discussed a greater number of topics, which was also associated with having a greater number of prenatal care visits.

Atherton, Feeg, and El-Adham (2004) conducted a study of epidural use using records of 2,355 women from the Agency for Healthcare Research and Quality (AHRQ) Medical Expenditure Panel Survey (MEPS) HC-046 (Pregnancy Files).

This dataset derives from a nationally representative survey of the U.S. civilian noninstitutionalized population. Researchers found that ethnicity was strongly associated with the nonuse of epidural procedures during normal vaginal deliveries, in that Hispanic women were found to be twice as likely as non-Hispanic women not to receive an epidural procedure. Race was coded as nonwhite or otherwise and ethnicity as Hispanic and otherwise; no mention was made of how ethnicity and race were determined. The authors concluded that "ethnicity rather than race [is] a culturally mediating variable in the likelihood to receive an epidural..." (Atherton, Feeg, and El-Adham, 2004: 11). This inappropriately appears to assume that homogeneity exists with regard to a specific feature across all Hispanic subgroups and/or that provider response to women who both self-identify as Hispanic and are perceived as Hispanic differs from their response to others.

Blackwell and colleagues (2004) conducted a study to identify the underlying genetic, developmental, and environmental risk factors for sudden infant death syndrome (SIDS) across three different ethnic groups with varying incidences of the syndrome: low, among Asians in Britain; moderate, among European/Caucasian groups; and high, among aboriginal Australians. The investigators reported that the major difference was the high levels of exposure to cigarette smoke among infants in the higher risk groups. The cigarette smoke was found to significantly reduce the anti-inflammatory cytokine interleukin-10 responses responsible for the pro-inflammatory responses that have been implicated in SIDS. In concluding that the examination "of the effects of genetic, developmental and environmental risk factors among different ethnic groups might be the key to future progress in understanding the causes of SIDS, rather than just the risk factors," (Blackwell, Moscovis, Gordon, Al Madani, Hall, Gleeson et al., 2004: 62) the authors recognized that ethnic differences are often clues, rather than answers in themselves.

Birth Outcomes

A Canadian study found that compared with white women, women of self-identified First Nations origin were at increased risk of neural tube defect-affected pregnancies (Ray, Vermeulen, Meier, Cole, and Wyatt, 2004). The risk of neural tube defect-affected pregnancy appeared to be similar among women of other self-identified ethnicities (Asian, black, other) compared to those who identified as white. The investigators advised that, if "the risk of NTD-affected pregnancies is truly higher among women of First Nations origin than among women of other origins, then the mechanisms for this discrepancy should be elucidated" (Ray, Vermeulen, Meuer, Cole, and Wyatt, 2004: 344), recognizing that it is not ethnicity *per se* that is determinative of any difference, should one actually exist. It is important to note that the category "First Nations" is not one that is used in the United States, although both countries claim native populations. Additionally, the categories that were used for ethnicity in this study frequently are used to delineate race in the United States, that is, white, black, Asian, and other.

Forrester and Merz (2003) relied on a population-based birth defects registry that included all Downs syndrome births delivered in Hawaii between 1986 and 2000 to calculate maternal age-specific Down syndrome rates for various racial and ethnic groups. Maternal race/ethnicity was classified for the purpose of this study into the following groups: Far East Asian (Japanese, Chinese, Korean); Pacific Islander (Hawaiian, Guamanian, Samoan), or Filipino. Women of other racial and ethnic groups were excluded because they represented 13% of all Down syndrome cases.

Investigators found that the rate of Down syndrome among Far East Asians and Filipinos was similar to whites where the maternal age was less than 35. However, among women age 35 and older, the rate of Down syndrome was lower for Pacific Islanders than for whites. The researchers advised that these findings were critical in order to better estimate a woman's risk of having an infant with Down syndrome. Other studies in Hawaii (Forrester and Merz, 2002; Forrester and Merz, 1999) and elsewhere have similarly found variations in rates of Down syndrome births across ethnic and racial groups (Centers for Disease Control and Prevention, 1994; Chavez, Cordero, and Becerra, 1988; Shaw, Carmichael, and Nelson, 2002), but such findings have not been consistent across all studies (Lau, Fung, Rogers, and Cheung, 1998).

Although various studies suggest that the rate of Down syndrome may vary across ethnic groups, it is unclear why, in this particular study, ethnicities were grouped as they were. No explanation is provided as to why Japanese, Chinese, and Korean are so similar as to warrant classification into the same category (Far East Asian) for the purpose of this analysis, or why Samoans, Guamanians, and Hawaiians similarly merit classification into one group. The investigators do not explain why Filipinos are so different from any of these groups as to warrant placement in a separate category. However, the answers to these questions may be critical to understanding how the investigators obtained the result that they did and the meaning of their findings if, indeed, the differences between groups exist.

Child Health and Disease

Various studies have reported differences in the rate of breastfeeding across ethnic/racial groups (Forste, Weiss, and Lippincott, 2001; Li and Grummer-Strawn, 2002; Li, Ogden, Ballew, Gillespie, and Grummer-Strawn, 2002; Li, Zao, Mokdad, Barker, and Grummer-Stawn, 2003). A more recent study conducted by Celi and colleagues (2005) utilized data from 1,829 women participating in a prospective cohort study of pregnant women and their children, known as Project Viva, to assess the relationship between race/ethnicity, immigration status, and social and economic factors on the initiation of breastfeeding. Race/ethnicity was determined by self-identification with one of the preformulated categories: Hispanic or Latina, white or Caucasian, black or African American, Asian or Pacific Islander, American Indian or Alaskan Native, and other. Individuals who self-identified as Asian, other, or who had missing race/ethnicity data were excluded from the analyses. "Cultural predictors" included country of origin, age at immigration, parental country of origin, and whether the individual was breastfed as an infant. "Social and economic predictors" referred to various sociodemographic factors, including education, income, and participant's age at delivery, among others.

The researchers found no significant difference in breastfeeding rates among U.S.-born women, regardless of their race or ethnicity. However, they indicated that immigrant women breastfed at significantly higher rates compared to U.S.-born women, even after adjustment for income level, educational level, and various other relevant factors. The authors concluded that "cultural factors, chiefly immigration status, were strongly associated with increased breastfeeding initiation in this cohort" (Celi, Rich-Edwards, Richardson, Kleinman, and Gillman, 2005).

A reliance on place of birth only as a marker of "cultural factors" assumes, first, that once an immigrant, always an immigrant; and, second, that there exists some level of similarity or homogeneity across all immigrant groups, regardless of their place of origin or length of residence outside of their countries of origin. It also ignores the variations that exist across immigration statuses with regard to the ability to access health care and health information outside of the study setting. The classification of individuals into the racial and ethnic categories as enumerated is also problematic. For instance, does a Latina with relatively lighter skin color self-classify as Latina or as white? Does a Caribbean Hispanic with darker skin self-classify as black or Hispanic? This lack of clarity with respect to the classification used results in confusion with regard to the interpretation of the findings.

Communicable Disease and Disease Risk

Researchers have estimated that there are currently 1,039,000 to 1,185,000 persons in the United States who are infected with HIV, and that approximately one-quarter of these individuals are unaware of their infection and diagnosis (Glynn and Rhodes, 2005). As of 2003, it was estimated that a total of 929,985 persons in the United States had an AIDS diagnosis and that, cumulatively, 524,060 individuals in the United States had died from HIV/AIDS since the beginning of the epidemic (Centers for Disease Control and Prevention, 2005). The Centers for Disease Control and Prevention (2005) has reported AIDS cases by race/ethnicity as follows:

TABLE 6. Estimated AIDS cases by race/ethnicity

Race or ethnicity	Estimated # of AIDS cases in 2003	Cumulative estimated # of AIDS cases, through 2003
White, not Hispanic	12,222	376,834
Black, not Hispanic	21,304	368,169
Hispanic	8,757	172,993
Asian/Pacific Islander	497	7,166
American Indian/Alaska Native	196	3,026

Researchers have frequently reported an association between risk behaviors and ethnicity in the context of HIV risk. As an example, Paxton and colleagues (2004) reported from their study of risk behaviors among European American, African American, and Hispanic women that "history of trauma, ethnicity, drug and alcohol use, homelessness, and being HIV-positive were associated with greater likelihood of engaging in high-risk sexual behaviors" (Paxton, Myers, Hall, and Javanbakht, 2004: 405), finding that being Latina or African American served as a protective factor in predicting the risk of engaging in risky sexual behavior. Various other factors, such as educational level and psychiatric disorder status, were not found to be predictive of sexual risk behavior. No explanation was offered as to the meaning of their conclusion regarding ethnicity which, as a risk factor, is not amenable to modification.

Similar concerns can be noted in a study conducted by Hickson and colleagues (2004) on HIV, sexual risk, and ethnicity among men in England who have sex with men (MSM). The authors concluded based on survey data gathered from 13,369 present in England that the higher HIV prevalence rate observed among black men in comparison with Asians and white British men was attributable to increased risk associated with higher levels of unprotected anal sex. The authors concluded that "HIV prevention programmes for MSM and African people should both prioritise black MSM" (Hickson, Reid, Weatherburn, Stephens, Nutland, and Boakye, 2004: 443). This conclusion, however, is unsupported by the data presented. If data were collected with respect to geographic region of origin or citizenship (for example, the Caribbean or Africa), those data were not presented. One must question, then, whether all individuals identified as black are to be considered African or whether only black Africans are to be considered at elevated risk. If this is the case, it is unclear why this distinction would be made based upon the data that were presented.

Researchers continue to utilize "race" and "ethnicity" synonymously, despite relative agreement in the literature regarding differences in their meaning. For instance, Apoola and colleagues (2005) in their study of treatment and partner notification outcomes for gonorrhea, conducted their analyses so that for "ethnicity purposes, those of black ethnicity were compared with non-blacks" although more detailed information pertaining to ethnicity had been collected from the study participants (Apoola, Mantella, Wotton, and Radcliffe, 2005: 287). No justification is provided for their decision to recode the ethnic data into these two groups and to equate skin color with ethnicity.

A similar lack of clarity in the use of the terms "ethnicity" and "race" are evident in a study of sexual partner choice among adolescents in the United States. The investigators sought to examine the relationship between individual-level demographic variables, community characteristics, and the characteristics of adolescents' sexual partners (Ford, Sohn, and Lepkowski, 2003). In describing the almost 8,000 respondents in the study, the researchers categorized them as white (62%), black (19.2%), Latino (11.7%), and other (7%) and referred to "variables Black ethnicity ... and Latino ethnicity" (Ford, Sohn, and Lepkowski, 2003: 214), failing to recognize that Latinos can be darker or lighter in skin color and that race and ethnicity are not interchangeable concepts. The authors concluded from their data that "the community characteristics of ethnic composition of the population and region were most strongly related to the ethnicity or race of the partner" (Ford, Sohn, and Lepkowski, 2003:216). It is unclear, however, whether they would have reached the same conclusion if race and ethnicity had not been collapsed in their analyses.

Similar issues arise in the context of public health functions. Public health surveillance activities frequently utilize race and ethnicity data to assist in tracking and preventing disease. However, the categories that are utilized in such efforts may be misleading and/or inadequate. As an example, investigators in Massachusetts attempted to obtain missing race/ethnicity information for STD morbidity reports that had been submitted through laboratories and diagnosing clinicians to the state (Chen, Etkind, Coman, Tang, and Whelan, 2003). The investigators indicated that, for the time period that was under study "race/ethnicity was reported as five mutually exclusive categories: white, black, Hispanic, Asian/Pacific Islander and Native American" (Chen, Etkind, Coman, Tang, and Whelan, 2003: 258). However, these categories are not mutually exclusive; individuals who claim Hispanic ethnicity may have darker or lighter skin tones, so that they may be identified as white or black. The investigators asserted that the collection of such data "is essential as a first step toward understanding the root causes of the disparities in the health status that are all too common in this nation" (Chen, Etkind, Coman, Tang, and Whelan, 2003: 262). However, presumably the primary function of surveillance is to identify those at risk of disease and to prevent disease transmission. Reliance on these broad categories would be inadequate to detect on a broader level networks within communities that could be associated with increased risk of transmission. For instance, classification of individuals as black would be inadequate to detect a pattern of transmission within networks of a particular ethnic enclave, such as inner city U.S.-born blacks or Caribbean blacks.

A report of a school-based hepatitis B immunization initiative also provokes thought as to the most appropriate approach to the classification of race and ethnicity. The author found that participation rates in the program "varied by race . . . with black and Hispanic potential enrollees participating more frequently than white and Asian potential enrollees" (Middleman, 2004: 414). Race, even if it is thought to exist as a social construct only, is inappropriately equated here with ethnicity.

A California-based study of differences in mortality among patients with community acquired pneumonia is instructive with respect to the care taken by the investigators to explain the limitations of their research and the meaning of their use of "race" and "ethnicity" as variables. Haas and colleagues (2003) examined the relationship between race/ethnicity and hospital characteristics and 30-day mortality, adjusting for clinical characteristics of the patients. Unfortunately, they categorized patients' ethnicity as white, African American, Hispanic, and Asian American, thereby equating race with ethnicity and failing to recognize, again, that Hispanics may have darker or lighter skin and consequently may be perceived as white or black. However, they presented the limitations of their findings—that Asian Americans experienced higher observed risk-adjusted mortality in public hospitals—in significant detail. The authors cautioned that (1) ethnicity had been determined from administrative data rather than self-report; (2) subgroup identity was unavailable; and (3) data relating to the process of care, the severity of illness, and the cause of death were unavailable. The authors concluded, further, that because their findings were inconsistent with their hypothesis, the results should be considered exploratory in nature.

Chronic Disease and Disease Risk

Obesity

Increasing attention has been focused on the existence of obesity and the establishment of healthy or unhealthy eating patterns in both children and adult populations. Americans appear to be eating more (Tippett and Cleveland, 1999) and consuming greater portions of food (Young and Nestle, 2002), including high-caloric, high fat fast food (Block, Scribner, and DeSalvo, 2004; Lin and Frazao, 1999; Massachusetts Medical Society Committee on Nutrition, 1989; Schlosser, 2001). Obesity has been found to increase the risk of various diseases, including cardiovascular disease, hypertension, Type II diabetes, and various types of cancer (Bray, Bouchard, and James, 1998). And, despite increased portion sizes, diets do not always reflect an intake of recommended vitamins and minerals that is adequate to prevent disease and maintain health. For instance, adequate calcium intake is believed to be critical for the development and maintenance of bone mass and reduce the risk of adult osteoporosis (Cromer and Harel, 2000), while an adequate intake of the vitamins derived from fresh fruits and vegetables is believed to be critical to the prevention of atherosclerosis, chronic respiratory diseases, and specific forms of cancer (Barker, 1997; McGill, Jr., McMahan, Malcom, Oalmann, and Strong, 1997; Steinmetz and Potter, 1991).

The Children's Health Study was a 10-year longitudinal study of the health effects of exposure to air pollution on school-age children residing in 12 communities within a 200-mile radius of Los Angeles (Xie, Gilliland, Li, and Rockett, 2003). Dietary information was collected from the participants beginning in 1998 and was used to investigate the overall nutritional status of adolescents between the ages of 11 and 20 and the effects of gender, ethnicity, family income, and education on the dietary patterns of these adolescents. Information on ethnicity and race was collected by self-report; categories were delineated as non-Hispanic white, Hispanic, African-American, Asian, and Other. Investigators concluded that (1) boys' intake of energy, protein, cholesterol, and calcium was higher than girls'; (2) girls' intake of carbohydrates, fiber, vitamin C, and vitamin A was higher than boys'; (3) Hispanics and Asians had a higher intake of cholesterol than did blacks and non-Hispanic whites; (4) calcium intake was greater among non-Hispanic whites and Hispanics than among blacks and Asians; (5) a higher proportion of non-Hispanic whites than other groups met the recommended daily allowances for intake of iron and folate.

Although these findings are helpful to some extent in identifying groups in which, as a group, there exists inadequate intake of nutritional requirements, the findings are also problematic. For instance, how were blacks classified if they did not self-identify as African-American, such as individuals who may have immigrated from Caribbean or African countries? As "Other?" If this is the case, is there sufficient homogeneity across all individuals within the category of "Other" to warrant placing them in the same category? For instance, are such individuals, if encompassed in that grouping, sufficiently similar to Native Americans to be grouped together with them? Hispanics of Caribbean origin have several categories from which to select their identity: Hispanic, African-American (if black and Hispanic), or Other. Inadequate information is provided in the text of the publication to enable the reader to determine the level of consistency across participants in their approach to this query or to determine the level of homogeneity across relevant characteristics of individuals within each category.

Similar difficulties are present, albeit perhaps to a lesser extent, in studies that relied on data from the National Health and Nutrition Examination Survey III (NHANES III), collected from 1988 to 1994. This database contains health information for 33,994 individuals from the United States' noninstitutionalized, civilian population aged 2 months and older (Zhang and Wang, 2003). A study by Zhang and Wang (2003), for instance, utilized data from 10,932 adults ages 18 to 60 to explore the relationship between socioeconomic status and obesity across sex, age, and ethnic subgroups. Based on self-reported ethnicity and race, individuals were classified for the purpose of this study as non-Hispanic white, non-Hispanic black, Mexican American, or Other. The authors reported an inverse relationship between socioeconomic status and obesity among non-Hispanic white men and women and all white gender-age groups, but a varying relationship between SES and obesity by gender and age among blacks and Mexican Americans. The authors noted that measures of SES may not be commensurate across various groups, rendering the findings more difficult to interpret and to utilize in practice. However, it is also possible that some individuals who were of Mexican ethnicity may have self-classified as "other" because they self-identified not as Mexican American, but as Chicano or Latino.

The difficulties inherent in this approach to the assessment of race and ethnicity can be contrasted with that utilized by Block and colleagues (2004) in their ecological study of the prevalence of fast food restaurants in various census tracts. This investigation involved the mapping of all fast food restaurants within the city limits of New Orleans, Louisiana and the identification of shopping areas in the relevant census tracts. Investigators assessed the association between fast food restaurant density in neighborhoods, controlling for levels of commercial activity, the presence of major highways, and median homes values, which were hypothesized to influence the placement of such restaurants. Neighborhoods were identified as predominantly black if, according to census data, 80% or more of their population was recorded as black. Although reliance on census categories is also somewhat problematic, it may be less so in view of the current ability of individuals to self-designate as black or African-American and to also designate whether or not they consider themselves to be Hispanic.

Diabetes

It has been estimated that more than 15 million Americans have a diagnosis of diabetes (Mokdad, Bowman, Ford, Vinicor, Mrks, and Koplan, 2001). Epidemiological data from various countries consistently suggest that the prevalence of diabetes is influenced by a large array of environmental and behavioral factors, including residence in rural versus urban areas (Kim, Kim, Lee, and Kim, 1976), migration to westernized nations from developing countries (McKeigue, Miller, and Marmot, 1989), level of physical activity (Manson, Rimm, Stampfer, Colditz, Willett, Krolewski et al., 1991), diet (Kudo, Falciglia, and Couch, 2000), and obesity (Sundquist and Winkleby, 2000). It has been argued, however, that factors such as obesity, fat distribution, level of exercise, or dietary intake do not by themselves account for observations of poorer gyclemic control among African Americans and Latinos (Auslander, Thompson, Dreitzer, White, and Santiago, 1997; Bond, Zaccaro, Karter, Selby, Saad, and Golff Jr., 2003; Eberhardt, Lackland, Wheeler, German, and Teutsch, 1994; Harris, Eastman, Cowie, Flegal, and Eberhardt, 1999; Saadine, Engelgau, Beckles, Gregg, Thompson, and Narayan, 2002; Weatherspoon, Kumanyika, Ludlow, and Schatz, 1994) and increased insulin resistance among Asian Indians in comparison with other ethnic groups (Chandalia, Abate, Garg, Stary-Gundersen, and Grundy, 1999) and genetic factors may play a more determinant role in the predisposition to diabetes (Abate and Chandalia, 2003).

Some researchers have questioned the appropriateness of relying on broad, ill-defined racial/ethnic categories in the context of studies relating to diabetes, while yet others have reported genetic evidence that supports categorization of race based on self-identification and have argued that reliance on such distinctions is appropriate for genetic studies (Risch, Burchard, Ziv, and Tang, 2002; Rosenberg, Pritchard, Weber, Cann, Kidd, Zhivotovsky, and Feldman, 2002). Still others have argued that delineation of individuals by race/ethnicity is critical in the context of diabetes prevention and control, not only because it will assist in the identification of those at higher risk, but also because dietary recommendations must be tailored to ethnic and cultural backgrounds in order to increase the likelihood of their acceptance by the populations involved (Abate and Chandalia, 2003; Franz, Bantle, Beebe, Brunzell, Chiasson, Garg, et al., 2002).

Breast Cancer

Breast cancer has been identified as "the most common invasive cancer in women" (Ghafoor, Jemal, Ward, Cokkinides, Smith and Thun, 2003) and, in the United States, is the most frequently diagnosed cancer in women ages 30 to 39 (Smith and Saslow, 2002) and the fourth most common cancer in women aged 20 to 29 (Ghafoor et al., 2003). Incidence rates are highest in industrialized nations, such as the United States, Western Europe, and Australia (Stewart and Kleihues, 2003). Various risk factors for breast cancer have been identified, including early age at menarche, later age at menopause, nulliparity or older age at first birth, lack or shorter-term breast-feeding, alcohol intake of one or more drinks per day, post-menopausal obesity, and long-term use of hormone replacement therapy (Henderson, Pike, Bernstein, and Ross, 1996; Kelsey and Bernstein, 1996; Ross, Paganini-Hill, Wan, and Pike, 2000). It is believed that these factors are surrogate measures of exposure to estrogen and possibly to progesterone (Bernstein, Teal, Joslyn, and Wilson, 2003).

In the United States, studies have consistently demonstrated advanced cancer stage at diagnosis, larger tumor size, unfavorable tumor biology, and/or poor ancillary health among African Americans with breast cancer as compared with white patients (Donegan and Tjoe, 2004; Chlebowski, Chen, Anderson, Rohan, Aragaki, Lane, et al., 2005; Elmore, Moceri, Carter, and Larson, 1998; Ghafoor, Jemal, Ward, Cokkinides, Smith and Thun, 2003; Li, Malone, and Daling, 2003). American Indians (Frost, Tollestrup, Hunt, Gilliland, Key, and Urbana, 1996; Sugarman, Dennis, and White, 1994) and Hispanic whites (Bentley, Delfino, Taylor, Howe, and Anton-Culver, 1998; Boyer-Chammard, Taylor, and Anton-Culver, 1999; Elledge, Clark, Chamness, and Osborne, 1994; Hsu, Glaser, and West, 1997; Zaloznik, 1997) have also been found to present with more advanced stages of breast cancer and, like African Americans, have poorer survival rates after diagnosis (Chevarley and White, 1997; Edwards, Gamel, Vaughan, and Wrightson, 1998; Joslyn and West, 2000).

This broad grouping of individuals, however, may be ill-advised. For instance, the groupings of "Hispanic" and "non-Hispanic" were created administratively in 1978 by the Office of Management and Budget and were accompanied by a cautionary note to refrain from interpreting them as scientific in nature (Fiellin, Chemerynski and Borak, 2003). Additionally, the North American Association of Central Cancer Registries has noted that

information about Hispanics/Latinos, the nation's fastest growing minority, is difficult to interpret because the data collection methods have not been uniformly applied, and have often not been well-defined. Even the terminology for referring to Hispanics may vary from region-region, and within a single area, from population-to-population (Office of Management and Budget, 1997).

Indeed, variations in risk have been reported across subgroups of broadly-defined ethnic and racial groups, underscoring the difficulty of subsuming individuals of varying backgrounds under one ethnic rubric. As an example, in comparison with non-Hispanic whites, it has been found that blacks, American Indians, Hawaiians, Asian Indians, Pakistanis, Mexicans, South and Central Americans, and Puerto Ricans have a greatly enhanced risk of presenting with stage IV breast cancer; blacks, Mexicans, and Puerto Ricans are more likely to receive or elect a first course of surgical and radiation treatment that does not meet the standards of the National Comprehensive Cancer network; and blacks, American Indians, Hawaiians, Vietnamese, Mexicans, South and Central Americans, and Puerto Ricans have an increased risk of mortality following breast cancer diagnosis (Li, Malone, and Daling, 2003). These subgroup variations have been hypothesized to result from differences in socioeconomic factors, patient-physician interactions, mammography use, obesity levels, tumor marker expression, and/or levels of knowledge (Li, Malone, and Daling, 2003). One research group concluded that

a combination of socioeconomic and lifestyle factors, and possibly tumor characteristics, are likely to contribute to the differences in stage at breast cancer presentation and survival rates by race and ethnicity. However, the differences in treatments received that [were] observed by race and ethnicity are likely to be solely the result of socioeconomic and cultural factors ((Li, Malone, and Daling, 2003: 56).

As with other diseases, it may be important to examine risk of disease and mortality from disease across perceived racial/ethnic groups in order to detect variations in health status and care that may be associated with discrimination (Krieger, Sidney, and Coakley, 1998; Tull and Chambers, 2001), variations in physician-patient interactions attributable to racial differences (van Ryn and Burke, 2000), barriers to care within groups of similarly-insured individuals (Karter, Ferrara, Darbinian, Ackerman, and Selby, 2000), and the impact of cumulative hardship (Lynch, Kaplan, and Shema, 1997). In examining factors such as the effects of racism on access to and level of health care, *perceived* race or ethnicity may be more relevant than even self-identified race or ethnicity, since it is the individual's perception that drives the interaction. In such instances, however, it is critical that data be collected on perceived identity of the patient by the provider, in addition to or instead of patient self-identity.

Smoking

Smoking is the leading cause of morbidity and mortality in the United States (Centers for Disease Control and Prevention, 1997; McGinnis and Foege, 1993). Smoking has been linked to cardiovascular disease, various forms of cancer, and chronic obstructive lung diseases (United States Department of Health and Human Services, 1990).

Smoking patterns in the United States have been shown to differ across socioeconomic and ethnic-gender groups. Data from the 2000 National Health Interview Survey indicate that there is a lower prevalence of smoking among Hispanics in comparison with non-Hispanic whites, African Americans, and Native Americans and a lower level of willingness to quit smoking (Trosclair, Husten, Pederson, and Dhillon, 2002). Research suggests that blacks begin smoking at a later age than whites (Centers for Disease Control and Prevention, 1997; Geronimus, Neidert, and Bound, 1993) and are less likely to quit smoking (McWhorter, Boyd, and Mattson, 1993; Novotny, Warner, Kendrick, and Remington, 1988; Wagenknecht, Maolio, Lewis, Perkins, Lando, and Hulley, 1993). Smoking prevalence among women is high (Centers for Disease Control and Prevention, 1999), and research suggests that women are less likely than men to quit smoking (Osler, Prescott, Godtfredsen, Hein, and Schnohr, 1999; Ward, Klesges, Zbikowski, Bliss, and Garvey, 1997; Wetter, Kenford, Smith, Fiore, Jorenby, and Baker, 1999). Since 1965, a greater proportion of white women than black women have ever smoked, average more cigarettes per day, and are more likely to be heavy smokers (United States Department of Health and Human Services, 2001). Black women have been found to be less likely than whites to attend smoking cessation groups (United States Department of Health and Human Services, 1998) and to quit smoking (Novotny, Warner, Kendrick, and Remington, 1988). Several studies have suggested that members of ethnic minority groups, and Hispanics in particular, are less likely to be advised by their health care providers to quit smoking (Denny, Serdula, Holtzman, and Nelson, 2003; Houston, Scarinci, Person, and Greene, 2005).

These observations regarding the prevalence of smoking, attempts to quit smoking, and success at such attempts across racial/ethnic groups may be confounded by various other factors. A study conducted by Barbeau, Krieger, and Soobader (2004) utilizing data from the 2000 National Health Survey Interview found that working class jobs, low educational level, and low income have been found to be independently associated with a higher prevalence of current smoking. Race and ethnicity were categorized in accordance with the 1997 Office of Management and Budget Directive 15: white, black, American Indian/Alaskan Native, Asian, and Hispanic (from any racial/ethnic group). The authors reported that information on nativity did not "materially affect" results of their multivariate models. However, one must wonder at the wisdom of including blacks born in the United States in a category with those born in other countries and encompassing in one group all individuals from Spanish-speaking countries, despite widely divergent norms and health practices; such a classification system assumes homogeneity within groups that are heterogeneous.

Mental Health

Many studies have reported disparities across racial and ethnic groups in the receipt of mental health services and the quality of the care received. However, neither the theoretical basis for the exploration of race/ethnicity nor the reasons for the manner in which these constructs are operationalized are always evident.

As an example, one research group examined the relationship between Hispanic ethnicity and the expression of complaints about antidepressant therapy among 98 patients, using audiotapes of physician-patient communication (Sleath, Rubin, and Wurst, 2003). The researchers reported that Hispanic patients expressed more complaints than did non-Hispanic whites. However, no explanation was offered as to why ethnicity might be associated with the frequency of such complaints.

In another study of mental health among Canadians, researchers concluded that East and Southeast Asians, Chinese, South Asians, and black Canadians have better mental health than English Canadians, who have better mental health than do Jewish Canadians (Wu, Noh, Kaspar, and Schimmelle, 2003). Researchers asked individuals two questions to assess race/ethnicity: "How would you best describe your race or colour?" and "To which ethnic or cultural group(s) did your ancestors belong?" Based on participants' responses, the investigators classified individuals into one of the following groups: East and Southeast Asian, Chinese, South Asian, Aboriginal, Black, Arabic and West Asian, Latin American, Jewish, French,

English, Other whites, and mixed racial groups. These categories unfortunately reflect a significant lack of clarity due to their overlapping nature. For instance, as but one example, Jews can be of Latin American, English, or French heritage and can be white or black. Additionally, the criteria used to delineate South Asians from East and Southeast Asians were unspecified, so that it is unclear what ethnicities are possibly encompassed within each label. As a result of these issues, the meaning and significance of the researchers' conclusions are questionable.

Another investigation that focused on medication adherence failed to adequately explain the differences reported in adherence across ethnic groups, although the data appear to have been available to do so, at least in part. Opolka and colleagues (2003) reported from their analysis of Texas Medicaid claims for persons who had been diagnosed with schizophrenia or schizoaffective disorder that African American and Hispanic patients were significantly less adherent than white patients. They also found, however, that patients were most adherent to olanzapine, followed by risperidone and haloperidol, and that nonwhite patients were less likely to be prescribed these latter two drugs, which appeared to have better tolerability and broader therapeutic efficacy (Frankenburg, 1999; Leucht, Pitschel-Walz, Abraham, and Kissling, 1999). It would not be implausible, then, to conclude that the lower rates of adherence may have been attributable to differences in prescribing patterns, rather than ethnicity *per se*, but the investigators did not address this possibility explicitly.

Intimate Partner Violence

It has been estimated that in the United States alone, each year approximately 4.4 million adult women are physically assaulted by their intimate partners (Plichta, 1997). One or both partners in approximately 500,000 couples sustain injuries from violence each year (Sorenson, Upchurch, and Shen, 1996). Women in the United States are at higher risk of homicide victimization than are women in any other high-income society (Hemenway, Shinoda-Tagawa, and Miller, 2002). In 1998, the deaths of almost three-quarters of all women murdered were attributable to their intimate partners (Rennison and Welchans, 2002). For the period 1993 through 1999, intimates killed 32% of all female murder victims ages 20 to 24 (Rennison, 2001). Additionally, homicide is a major contributor to deaths occurring during pregnancy (Dannenberg, Carter, Lawson, et al., 1995).

Women who appear to be at highest risk of assault by intimate partners are younger, urban dwellers, African Americans, and those with lesser education and lower incomes (Sorenson, Upchurch, and Shen, 1996). Women under the age of 20 are more likely to know their assailant as an acquaintance than are older women (Peipert and Domagalstei, 1994). Women who receive what had been known as Aid to Families with Dependent Children ("welfare") were found to be three times as likely to have experienced partner aggression during the previous year than were non-recipient women (Corlett, 1999).

Female victims of intimate partner violence have been found more likely to use multiple substances (cigarettes, alcohol, and illegal drugs) than are nonvictims

(Martin, English, Clark, Silenti, and Kupper, 1996). This association has been found in the context of dating violence (Makepeace, 1981). Partner violence often begins or escalates during pregnancy (Gillespie, 1988); pregnant women especially at risk for violence during their pregnancies are those who have been battered prior to pregnancy (McFarlane, Parker, Soeken, and Bullock, 1992). A study of AFDC women in Massachusetts suggested an increased risk of abuse directed towards women who bore and cared for a disabled child (Corlett, 1999). Homicide has been found more likely to occur among couples of lower socioeconomic status (Chimbos, 1998) and those in which the wife is substantially younger than the husband (Chimbos, 1998; Cohen, Llorente, and Eisdorfer, 1998).

Research suggests that within the United States, the frequency of partner violence varies across subgroups. However, many of these studies often fail to specify how ethnicity and/or race are determined in the context of the study and, if such variations do, indeed, exist, insufficient research has been conducted to establish the reasons for these differences.

A study by Cazenave and Straus (1979) found that within a nationally representative sample of African-Americans and non-Hispanic whites, the rates of intimate partner violence were lower among the African-Americans in 3 of 4 income strata, after controlling for race, income, and occupation. They also found that women were less likely to be assaulted if they had a strong family and social network. Hispanic women have been found to be at greater risk of physical violence during marriage as compared with women of other ethnic groups (Straus and Smith, 1990). These findings stand in contrast to those of other studies that have consistently found that the rates of partner violence are similar across racial and/or ethnic groups (Gondolf, Fisher, and McFerron, 1988; Lockhart and White, 1989; Stark, 1990).

A number of studies have found that even when the rates of violence are similar *across* racial/ethnic groups, the experience of partner violence may differ. For instance, several research groups have found that in comparison with non-Hispanic white women, Hispanic women are more likely to have been the victims of violence for a longer period of time (Gondolf, Fisher, and McFerron, 1988; Torres, 1991). The level of violence suffered by African-American women at the hands of their partners has been found to be more lethal than that among non-Hispanic whites, even though the incidence rates are similar (Stark, 1990).

One of the difficulties with such studies is the underlying assumption of homogeneity within broadly framed ethnic classifications. For instance, such studies assume that there are greater commonalities across all Hispanic subgroups in comparison with subgroups of Hispanics and subgroups of other groups, such as non-Hispanic whites or African-Americans. We do not know, however, whether this actually holds true in this context. Additionally, researchers may speak of race and ethnicity as if they are interchangeable concepts, which they are not. For instance, one study of physical abuse during and after pregnancy examined "ethnicity" as a risk factor among individuals classified as African American, white, Mexican and Mexican American, Cuban American, Puerto Rican, or Central American (Bohn, Tebben, and Campbell, 2004), although whites are of diverse ethnicities and individuals with darker skin may be neither African American nor of any form of Latino heritage.

For instance, several studies that have examined partner violence across sub-groups of larger ethnic classifications have found that the frequency of violence may vary even *within* United States subgroups. One study found that, although a smaller proportion of African-American women in upper socioeconomic strata report partner violence, they report a higher median number of assaults per year in comparison with African-American women in lower socioeconomic strata. It has been reported that Puerto Rican husbands are 10 times as likely as Cuban husbands to assault their wives (Kantor, Jasinski, and Aldarondo, 1994). Compared to non-Hispanic whites and U.S.-born Mexican-Americans, Mexican-born Mexican-Americans have reported lower rates of partner violence (Sorenson and Telles, 1991). Several research groups have reported that factors such as immigration status, prejudice, a lack of English proficiency, and the lack of emotional support resulting from separation from extended families may contribute to the abuse (Ho, 1990; Perilla, Bakeman, and Norris, 1994).

Despite our knowledge relating to the incidence and prevalence of partner violence and risk factors for partner violence, we actually have relatively little knowledge about how partner violence is viewed within various groups, both within and outside of the United States. One of the few United States studies to examine diverse perspectives found that compared to non-Hispanic white women, Mexican-American women are less likely to classify behavior such as slapping, pushing, shoving, grabbing, and throwing things at them as physical abuse (Torres, 1991). Puerto Ricans appear to have the highest rate of cultural approval of wife assaults as compared to non-Hispanic whites, Cubans, and Mexican-Americans (Kantor et al., 1994), although the reasons for this difference have not been investigated.

A recent ethnography of low-income, predominantly second generation, mainland Puerto Rican adolescents found that both males and females condone the use of physical violence as a punishment for females who were perceived to be sluts, that is, those whose sexual behavior was seen as being similar to males (Asencio, 1999). Females could have intercourse without becoming sluts only if they were truly in love. Accordingly, females who left relationships "too early" or had not sacrificed sufficiently to preserve the relationship were suspected of having engaged in sex out of lust and not out of love. As a result, females often stayed in abusive relationships to protect their reputations and to avoid further violence. In addition, some males believed that a female could not leave a relationship until the male gave her permission to do so. If the female left the relationship and was with a new male partner, she was potentially subject to physical violence from her former partner because she had become a slut (Asencio, 1999).

Sex and Sexual Orientation in Health Research

In contrast to the frequent inclusion of ethnicity and race as variables in health research, and the inclusion, as well, of biological sex as a variable to be addressed, there has been a notable lack of attention to issues pertaining to gender, gender role, and sexual orientation. Unfortunately, this too often occurs even in contexts in which one or more of these variables may be highly relevant, such as studies that focus on sexual behavior and disease transmission, on child rearing practices, and illness behaviors, to name but a few. Additionally, many of the methodological issues that are associated with the use of race and ethnicity data in the conduct and reporting of research are also reflected in studies that focus on sex role and sexual orientation.

This discussion focuses on the operationalization of sexual orientation in a variety of studies and the strengths and weaknesses of each approach. In assessing each approach, it may be helpful to recall that sexual orientation is a multi-dimensional construct; that sexual orientation may be fluid throughout one's lifetime; that how an individual identifies him- or herself may or may not reflect the sex of his or her sexual partners as may be the case, for instance, with individuals who self-identify as homosexual but have sexual relations with both men and women; and that self-identification as having a particular sexual orientation may precede or post-date actual sexual relations.

Communicable Disease and Disease Risk

Researchers conducting a study of contact tracing for gonorrhea examined the effectiveness of the practice in conjunction with sexual orientation in men (Rogstad, Clementson, and Ahmed-Jushuf (1999). They concluded that Caucasian gay men had a higher mean number of sexual contacts as compared with white heterosexual men. However, the authors failed to specify how they assessed sexual orientation. If self-identity was utilized, it is also possible that individuals who self-identified as heterosexual may have had sexual relations with other men that remained unreported.

Schindhelm and Hospers (2004) investigated the relation between sexual activity and sexual risk-taking behavior among men prior to "coming out." They found that individuals who had sex with men before coming out had more lifetime sex partners and more casual sex partners during the preceding six months, and that a greater proportion of these men engaged in unsafe sex practices. Their assessment of sexual orientation was considerably more explicit than that of the previously mentioned study. Individuals were asked to place themselves on a five-point scale that ranged from *completely heterosexual* to *completely homosexual* and to utilize yet another scale to indicate their level of self-acceptance. This approach permitted the classification of individuals in a manner consistent with their self-identity. However, it is also possible that variation existed across study participants. For instance, one might have assessed his orientation based upon desired sexual acts only, while yet another may have also considered instances of survival sex or coerced sex, and yet another may have factored in emotional intimacy with either sex as a component of his orientation.

Wold and colleagues (1998) assessed the prevalence of unsafe sex in bisexual and gay men. Men were classified as bisexual if they had had sex with at least one man and at least one women in the previous six months, and were classified as homosexual if they had had sexual relations with only men during that period of time. All of the participants were recruited from explicitly gay venues for a study of risk behaviors in gay men. Consequently, it is possible that many, if not most or all, of the participants self-identified as gay, even though some had had sexual relations with one or more women. The authors unfortunately used the terms "homosexual/gay" and "bisexual" interchangeably with the terms "homosexually active men" and "bisexually active men," thereby confusing issues of identity with issues of behavior.

Chronic Disease and Disease Risk

The incidence of cancer of the anal canal, which extends from the upper to the border of the anal sphincter, is relatively low (Gervaz, Allal, Villiger, Bühler, and Morel, 2003), constituting just 1.5% of all digestive cancers in the United States. The United States has an estimated 3,400 new cases each year in the United States and 500 deaths recorded from the disease in 1999 (Greenlee, Murray, Bolden, and Wingo, 2000; Ryan, Compton, and Mayer, 2000). Research findings strongly suggest an association between receptive anal intercourse and the development of anal cancer (Bjorge, Engeland, Luostarinen, Mork, Gislefoss et al., 2002; Frisch, Glimelius, van den Brule, Wohlfart, Meijer et al., 1997). Risk factors for the disease in women include a history of multiple sexual partners, a history of anal warts, and anal intercourse before the age of 30 (Frisch, Glimelius, van den Brule, Wohlfart, Meijer et al., 1997).

Gervaz and colleagues (2003) authored an excellent review of the research relating to the pathogenesis and treatment of anal cancer. However, despite research findings indicating that receptive anal sex appears to be a risk factor for anal cancer, regardless of the sex of the individual, they concluded that "cytological screening of male homosexuals with an anal Papanicolaou test may help in identifying high-grade dysplasia and preventing anal cancer" (Gervaz et al., 2003: 353). This conclusion assumes, incorrectly, that most, if not all, male homosexuals engage in receptive anal intercourse. It further creates the impression that women who engage in receptive anal intercourse are not at risk of the disease. Unfortunately, the recommendation focused on sexual orientation, rather than the sexual behavior that past research findings implicate as a risk factor.

A study conducted by Matthews' research team (2002) investigated cancer experiences, medical interactions related to cancer treatment, and quality of life among a sample of heterosexual women and lesbians. The researchers reported that lesbians experienced higher stress levels in association with their diagnosis and lower levels of satisfaction with the care received. To determine lesbian status or heterosexuality, individuals were asked to complete a self-report, in which they indicated their sexual orientation. Lesbians were then asked another series of questions relating to the extent to which they had disclosed their sexual orientation to others. It appears that classification as a lesbian or heterosexual was made entirely on the basis of self-identification. However, the criteria used by respondents to self-identify and the meaning of those criteria may have varied across respondents. For instance, some women may have self-identified as lesbian and never have had sexual relations with men, while others may have actually had more sexual encounters with men than with women, or may have been involved sexually with one or more men for longer periods of time than with women. It is unclear whether or to what extent misclassification may have occurred due to lack of clarity in the classification criteria and to what extent they may have affected the findings.

Similar concerns can be detected in a study of breast cancer incidence among lesbian women and their heterosexual sisters conducted by Dibble and colleagues (2004). In this study, the researchers recruited lesbian women through a variety of lesbian-friendly venues. Although the researchers acknowledged that varying definitions of lesbian status are utilized, they relied solely upon respondent self-identification as lesbian, without collection of data on sexual behaviors. Because this study explicitly included heterosexual women as well as lesbians, it is possible that some of the women who self-identified as heterosexual may have had relationships with women and may have exactly the same behavioral profile as some of the self-identified lesbian respondents.

Self-identification was utilized as a basis for determining eligibility for participation in a study of disclosure of lesbian sexual orientation to physicians by lesbians with breast carcinoma (Boehmer and Case, 2004). Researchers targeted in their recruitment efforts "sexual minority" women, which they defined as "stating a lesbian or bisexual identity and included women who reported partnering with women, in an attempt to be inclusive of women who might feel uncomfortable embracing a lesbian or bisexual identity" (Boehmer and Case, 2004: 1883). This operationalization of sexual orientation appropriately focused on the behavior that was implicated by the research question, rather than an identity.

Mental Health

A review of earlier writings related to mental health and illness reveals significant confusion in the professional literature regarding the nature of sexual orientation and mental illness. Cameron (1963), for instance, reported that male schizophrenics evidence "feminine" characteristics on the left parts of their bodies, while female schizophrenics displayed "male" characteristics on their right. He attributed this to identification in schizophrenic thinking of the left side with femininity and the right side with masculinity.

Studies have consistently reported elevated rates of depression, mood disorders, substance use disorders, suicidal ideation, and completed suicide among gay/lesbian and bisexual children and adults in comparison with their heterosexual counterparts (Bagley and Tremblay, 1997; Cochran and Mays, 2000a,b; Faulkner and Cranston, 1998; Garofalo, Wolf, Wissow et al., 1999). A cross-sectional study conducted in Australia among 4,824 adults of two different age groups concluded that a higher prevalence of anxiety, depression existed among those who self-identified as bisexuals in comparison with self-identified heterosexuals, who had the lowest prevalence, and homosexuals, who fell between the other two groups. Both bisexuals and homosexuals reported greater childhood adversity and less positive family support than did heterosexuals. Sexual orientation was assessed in this study based on respondents' answer to a single question: "Would you currently consider yourself to be predominantly: heterosexual, homosexual, bisexual, don't know?" Because the study utilized a cross-sectional design and focused on currently-identified sexual orientation and mental status, it is impossible to know if the reported depression and anxiety occurred prior to a realization of identity or if it post-dated it. Additionally, because the question focused on self-identification only, without regard to behavior, it is impossible to assess the interplay, if any, between specific patterns of behavior and the mental health symptoms. For example, perhaps depression is more strongly associated with having multiple partners due to the lack of a stable relationship. Conversely, it might be associated with not having any partner because of a feeling of isolation.

Stigmatization

Numerous studies have examined attitudes towards homosexuals and lesbians (Heaven, 1999; Herek, 1984; Hinrichs and Rosenberg, 2002; Kite and Whitley, 1998; Lippincott, Wlazelek, and Schumacher, 2000). One such study investigated attitudes of female heterosexual university students of varying ethnicities towards homosexuals (Span and Vidal, 2003). The investigators found from their data that Asian students evidenced more homophobia than did Hispanic and Caucasian students. The study did not examine, however, individuals' conceptualizations of what a "homosexual" is, so that it is impossible to know if student-respondents were thinking of the same behaviors or characteristics in responding to the questions. For instance, some individuals may have answered based upon their vision of sexual intercourse between two men, while others may have focused on behaviors that they considered effeminate. Additionally, sexual orientation of the respondents was based on self-reported identity, not on behavior. It is possible, therefore, that some of the respondents themselves may have had same-sex romantic/sexual relationships, and that these experiences may be relevant to their expressed attitudes. The investigators appeared to equate self-identified race/ethnicity with culture, explaining that a "variable that has received little attention in this literature on homophobia is culture" (Span and Vidal, 2003: 565). Earlier discussion in this text refutes the assumption that these constructs are synonyms for each other.

Cameron, Landess, and Cameron (2005) compared individuals who acknowledged having engaged in "homosexual sex," illegal drug users, participants in prostitution, and smokers against individuals who abstained from these behaviors, using data derived from the National Household Survey on Drug Abuse. They concluded that homosexuals were more frequently disruptive, were less frequently productive, and generated excessive costs to society. They further concluded on the basis of their comparison of subsamples of homosexuals and blacks that societal discrimination did not explain these differences because these behavioral markers occurred at differing frequencies in these two groups. "Homosexuality" for the purpose of their analyses was determined by respondents' disclosure of having had same-sex sexual activity within the previous 12 months.

Numerous methodological difficulties are associated with this study. First, same-sex sexual activity may or may not be indicative of sexual orientation, as previously noted. Consequently, some of the individuals who were classified in the study as homosexual may, in fact, not consider themselves homosexual for any number of reasons. They may usually have sexual relations with a woman, but have been involved on limited occasions with a man, for instance, to experiment with their own sexuality or in exchange for shelter or while in prison. Second, the behavioral categories used to classify individuals clearly overlap: individuals who engage in prostitution may also smoke and may also use drugs, regardless of their sexual orientation. It is unclear how the researchers categorized individuals who had multiple behaviors. Finally, a number of the other comparisons made suffer from the same weakness. For instance, the behaviors of homosexuals are compared to those of blacks. However, some homosexuals are black. Were these individuals excluded from the analysis? Categorized as black? Categorized as homosexual?

Two of the same researchers, Cameron and Cameron (1996) conducted a study with 5,182 adults to assess the effect of a teacher's homosexuality on the development of homosexuality in the respondents. Respondents were asked to indicate whether they considered their sexual orientation at the time of the study to be heterosexual, homosexual, or bisexual; whether they had ever had a sexual experience with a heterosexual teacher or a homosexual teacher; whether a teacher had ever made "serious" sexual advances towards them; and the degree to which they believed that the teacher influenced them "to try homosexuality." The authors concluded that homosexuals more frequently claimed to have had homosexual teachers and more frequently reported homosexual sex with teachers. They further argued that these findings supported the contagion model of homosexuality, that is, that homosexuality is "taught or caught by sexual interaction with homosexual practitioners" (Cameron and Cameron, 1996: 603).

As with the previous study, there are critical methodological difficulties with their analyses. First, they relied on self-reported sexual orientation as a measure of homosexuality, despite the complexity of the construct. Consequently, some of the individuals who self-reported homosexual orientation may, in fact, have had sexual encounters with members of the opposite sex, and individuals who claimed a heterosexual orientation may have engaged in sexual relations with members of the same sex. Second, the researchers were actually measuring the students' perception of homosexuality/heterosexuality in their teachers; there is no way to verify whether, in fact, the teachers to whom respondents attributed a homosexual or heterosexual orientation would actually claim such orientation for themselves. In addition, the investigators fail to distinguish between sexual orientation, whether heterosexual or homosexual, and pedophilia, which involves sexual predation of children and is independent of sexual orientation (Loue, 2006).

Summary

This brief review of health research findings related to race, ethnicity, and sexual orientation underscores the importance of delineating specifically the research population and of avoiding an assumption of homogeneity within and across groups. It is critical that researchers explain what they mean by race and ethnicity and why they have used these constructs to describe their research populations and to frame their findings. The labels used to describe groups are often not synonymous with the behavior of interest and a failure to distinguish between them may lead to misleading and erroneous conclusions.

References

Abate, N., Chandalia, M. (2003). The impact of ethnicity on type 2 diabetes. *Journal of Diabetes and Its Complications* 17: 39–58.

Apoola, A., Mantella, I., Wotton, M., Radcliffe, K. (2005). Treatment and partner notification outcomes for gonorrhoea: Effect of gender and ethnicity. *International Journal of STD & AIDS* 16: 287–289.

Asencio, M.W. (1999). Machos and sluts: Gender, sexuality, and violence among a cohort of Puerto Rican adolescents. *Medical Anthropology Quarterly* 13(1): 107–126.

Atherton, M.J., Feeg, V.D., El-Adham, A.F. (2004). Race, ethnicity, and insurance as determinants of epidural use: Analysis of a national sample survey. *Nursing Economics* 22(1): 6–12.

Auslander, W.F., Thompson, S., Dreitzer, D., White, N.H., Santiago, J.V. (1997). Disparity in glycemic control and adherence between African-American and Caucasian youths with diabetes: Family and community contexts. *Diabetes Care* 20: 1569–1575.

Bagley, C., Trenblay, P. (1997). Suicidal behaviors in homosexual and bisexual males. *Crisis* 18: 24–34.

Barbeau, E.M., Krieger, N., Soobader, M.J. (2004). Working class matters: Socioeconomic disadvantage, race/ethnicity, gender, and smoking in NHIS 2000. *American Journal of Public Health* 94(2): 269–278.

Barker, D.J. (1997). Maternal nutrition, fetal nutrition, and disease in later life. *Nutrition* 13(9): 807–813.

Barr, D.A. (2004). Race/ethnicity and patient satisfaction: Using the appropriate method to test for perceived difference in race. *Journal of General Internal Medicine* 19(9): 937–943.

Bentley, J.R., Delfino, R.J., Taylor, T.H., Howe, S., Anton-Culver, H. (1998). Differences in breast cancer stage at diagnosis between non-Hispanic white and Hispanic populations, San Diego County, 1988–1993. *Breast Cancer Research and Treatment* 50: 1–9.

Bernstein, L., Teal, C.R., Joslyn, S., Wilson, J. (2003). Ethnicity-related variation in breast cancer risk factors. *Cancer* 97(1 Suppl.): 222–229.

Bjorge, T., Engeland, A., Luostarinen, T., Mork, J., Gislefoss, R.E. et al. (2002). Human papillomavirus infection as a risk factor for anal and perianal skin cancer in a prospective study. *British Journal of Cancer* 87: 61–64.

Blackwell, C.C., Moscovis, S.M., Gordon, A.E., Al Madani, O.M., Hall, S.T., Gleeson, M. et al. (2004). Ethnicity, infection, and sudden infant death syndrome. *FEMS Immunology and Medical Microbiology* 42(1): 53–65.

Bliss, E.B., Meyers, D.S., Phillips, Jr., R.L., Fryer, G.E., Dovey, S.M., Green, L.A. (2004). Variation in participation in health care settings associated with race and ethnicity. *Journal of General Internal Medicine* 19(9): 931–936.

Block, J.P., Scribner, R.A., DeSalvo, K.B. (2004). Fast food, race/ethnicity, and income: A geographic analysis. *American Journal of Preventive Medicine* 27(3): 211–217.

Boehmer, U., Case, P. (2004). Physicians don't ask, sometimes patients tell: Disclosure of sexual orientation among women with breast carcinoma. *Cancer* 101: 1882–1889.

Bohn, D.K., Tebben, J.G., Campbell, J.C. (2004). Influences of income, education, age, and ethnicity on physical abuse before and during pregnancy. *Journal of Obstetric, Gynecologic, and Neonatal Nursing* 33(5): 561–571.

Bonds, D.E., Zaccaro, D.J., Karter, A.J., Selby, J.V., Saad, M., Golff, D.C., Jr. (2003). Ethnic and racial differences in diabetes care: The Insulin Resistance Atherosclerosis study. *Diabetes Care* 26: 1040–1046.

Boyer-Chammard, A., Taylor, T.H., Anton-Culver, H. (1999). Survival differences in breast cancer among racial/ethnic groups: A population-based study. *Cancer Detection and Prevention* 23: 463–473.

Bray, G.A., Bouchard, C., James, W.P.T. (1998). *Handbook of Obesity*. New York: Marcel Dekker.

Cameron, N. (1963). *Personality Development and Psychopathology*. Boston, Massachusetts: Houghton Mifflin Company.

Cameron, P., Cameron, K. (1996). Do homosexual teachers pose a risk to pupils? The *Journal of Psychology* 130(6): 603–613.

Cameron, P., Landess, T., Cameron, K. (2005). Homosexual sex as harmful as drug abuse, prostitution, or smoking. *Psychological Reports* 96(3): 915–961.

Cazenave, N.A., Straus, M.A. (1979). Race, class, network embeddedness and family violence: A search for potent support systems. *Journal of Comparative Family Studies* 10: 280–300.

Celi, A.C., Rich-Edwards, J.W., Richardson, M.K., Kleinman, K.P., Gillman, M.W. (2005). Immigration, race/ethnicity, and social and economic factors as predictors of breastfeeding initiation. *Archives of Pediatric and Adolescent Medicine* 159: 255–260.

Centers for Disease Control and Prevention. (1999). Cigarette smoking among adults—United States, 1997. *Morbidity and Mortality Weekly Reports* 48: 993–996.

Centers for Disease Control and Prevention. (1994). Down syndrome prevalence at birth—United States, 1983–1990. *Morbidity and Mortality Weekly Reports* 43: 617–622.

Centers for Disease Control and Prevention. (1997). Smoking-attributable mortality and years of potential life lost—United States, 1984. *Morbidity and Mortality Weekly Report* 46: 444–451.

Centers for Disease Control and Prevention, National Center for HIV, STD, and TB Prevention. (2005). Basic Statistics. Available at http://www.cdc.gov/hiv/stats.htm#hivest. Last accessed December 7, 2005.

Chavez, G.F., Cordero, J.F., Becerra, J.E. (1988). Leading major congenital malformations among minority groups in the United States, 1981–1986. *Morbidity and Mortality Weekly Report CDC Surveillance Summary* 37: 17–24.

Chen, J., Etkind, P., Coman, G., Tang, Y., Whelan, M. (2003). Eliminating missing race/ethnicity data from a sexually transmitted disease case registry. *Journal of Community Health* 28(4): 257–265.

Chevarley, F., White, E. (1997). Recent trends in breast cancer mortality among white and black US women. *American Journal of Public Health* 87: 775–781.

Chimbos, P.D. (1998). Spousal homicides in contemporary Greece. International *Journal of Contemporary Sociology* 39: 213–223.

Chlebowski, R.T., Chen, Z., Anderson, G.L., Rohan, T., Aragaki, A., Lane, D., Doan, N.C., Paskett, E.D., McTiernan, A., Hubbell, F.A., Adams-Campbell, L.L., Prentice, R. (2005). Ethnicity and breast cancer: Factors influencing differences in incidence and outcome. *Journal of the National Cancer Institute* 97(6): 439–448.

Clark, T., Sleath, B., Rubin, R.H. (2003). Influence of ethnicity and language concordance on physician-patient agreement about recommended changes in public health behavior. *Patient Education and Counseling* 53(1): 87–93.

Cochran, S.D., Mays, V.M. (2000a). Lifetime prevalence of suicide symptoms and affective disorders among men reporting same-sex sexual partners: Results from NHANES III. *American Journal of Public Health* 90: 573–578.

Cochran, S.D., Mays, V.M. (2000b). Relation between psychiatric syndromes and behaviorally defined sexual orientation in a sample of the US population. *American Journal of Epidemiology* 151: 516–523.

Cohen, D., Llorente, M. & Eisdorfer, C. (1998). Homicide-suicide in older persons. *American Journal of Psychiatry* 155: 390–396.

Corlett, J.R. (1999, June 9). Women, domestic violence, and welfare. *Human Services Agenda of Northeast Ohio* 3: 105.

Dannenberg, A.L., Carter, D.M., Lawson, H.W. et al. (1995). Homicide and other injuries as causes of maternal deaths in New York City, 1987 through 1991. *American Journal of Obstetrics and Gynecology* 172: 1557–1564.

Denny, C.H., Serdula, M.K., Holtzman, D., Nelson, D.E. (2003). Physician advice about smoking and drinking: Are US adults being informed? *American Journal of Preventive Medicine* 24(1): 71–74.

Dibble, S.L., Roberts, S.A., Nussey, B. (2004). Comparing breast cancer risk between lesbian and their heterosexual sisters. *Women's Health Issues* 14: 60–68.

Donegan, W.L., Tjoe, J.A. (2004). Jewish ethnicity and black race: Contrasting influences on the prognosis of breast cancer. *Journal of Surgical Oncology* 87(2): 61–67.

Eberhardt, M.S., Lackland, D.T., Wheeler, F.C., German, R.R., Teutsch, S.M. (1994). Is race related to glycemic control? An assessment of glycosylated hemoglobin in two South Carolina communities. *Journal of Clinical Epidemiology* 47: 1181–1189.

Edwards, M.J., Gamel, J.W., Vaughan, W.P., Wrightson, W.R. (1998). Infiltrating ductal carcinoma of the breast: The survival impact of race. *Journal of Clinical Oncology* 16: 2693–2699.

Elledge, R.M., Clark, G.M., Chamness, G.C., Osborne, C.K. (1994). Tumor biologic factors and breast cancer prognosis among white, Hispanic, and black women in the United States. *Journal of the National Cancer Institute* 86: 705–712.

Elmore, J.G., Moceri, V.M., Carter, D., Larson, E.B. (1998). Breast carcinoma tumor characteristics in black and white women. *Cancer* 83: 2509–2515.

Faulkner, A.H., Cranston, K. (1998). Correlates of same-sex sexual behavior in a random sample of Massachusetts high school students. *American Journal of Public Health* 88: 262–266.

Felix-Aaron, K., Moy, E., Kang, M., Patel, M., Chesley, F.D., Clancy, C. (2005). Variation in quality of men's health care by race/ethnicity and social class. *Medical Care* 43(3 Suppl.): I-72–I-81.

Fiellin, M., Chemerynski, S., Borak, J. (2003). Race, ethnicity, and the SEER database. *Medical and Pediatric Oncology* 41: 413–414.

Ford, K., Sohn, W., Lepkowski, J.M. (2003). Ethnicity or race, area characteristics, and sexual partner choice among American adolescents. *The Journal of Sex Research* 40(2): 211–218.

Forrester, M.B., Merz, R.D. (2002). Epidemiology of Down syndrome (trisomy 21), Hawaii, 1986–97. *Teratology* 65: 207–212.

Forrester, M.B., Merz, R.D. (2003). Maternal age-specific Down syndrome rates by maternal race/ethnicity, Hawaii, 1986–2000. *Birth Defects Research (Part A)* 67: 625–629.

Forrester, M.B., Merz, R.D. (1999). Prenatal diagnosis and elective termination of Down syndrome in a racially mixed population in Hawaii, 1987–1996. *Prenatal Diagnosis* 19: 136–141.

Frankenburg, F.R. (1999). Choices in antipsychotic therapy in schizophrenia. *Harvard Review of Psychiatry* 6: 241–249.

Franz, M.J., Bantle, J.P., Beebe, C.A., Brunzell, J.D., Chiasson, J.L., Garg, A., Holzmeister, L.A., Hoogwerf, B., Mayer-Davis, E., Mooradian, A.D., Purnell, J.Q., Wheeler, M. (2002). Evidence-based nutrition principles and recommendations for the treatment and prevention of diabetes and related complications. *Diabetes Care* 25: 148–198.

Frisch, M., Glimelius, B., van den Brule, A.J.C., Wohlfart, J., Meijer, C.J. et al. (1997). Sexually transmitted infection as a cause of anal cancer. *New England Journal of Medicine* 337: 1350–1358.

Frost, F., Tollestrup, K., Hunt, W.C., Gilliland, F., Key, C.R., Urbina, C.E. (1996). Breast cancer survival among New Mexico Hispanic, American Indian, and non-Hispanic white women (1973–1992). *Cancer Epidemiology Biomarkers Prevention* 4: 861–866.

Garofalo, R., Wolf, C., Wissow, L.S., Woods, E.R., Goodman, E. (1999). Sexual orientation and risk of suicide attempts among a representative sample of youth. *Archives of Pediatric and Adolescent Medicine* 155(3): 487–493.

Geronimus, A.T., Neidert, L.J., Bound, J. (1993). Age patterns of smoking in U.S. black and white women of childbearing age. *American Journal of Public Health* 83: 1258–1264.

Gervaz, P., Allal, A.S., Villiger, P., Bühler, L., Morel, P. (2003). Squamous cell carcinoma of the anus: Another sexually transmitted disease. *Swiss Medical Weekly* 133: 353–359.

Ghafoor, A., Jemal, A., Ward, E., Cokkinides, V., Smith, R., Thun, M. (2003). Trends in breast cancer by race and ethnicity. *CA: A Cancer Journal for Clinicians* 53: 342–355.

Glynn M., Rhodes P. (2005). Estimated HIV prevalence in the United States at the end of 2003. Presented at the National HIV Prevention Conference, June; Atlanta [Abstract 595].

Gondolf, E.W., Fisher, E., McFerron, J.R. (1988). Racial differences among shelter residents: A comparison of Anglo, black, and Hispanic battered women. *Journal of Family Violence* 3: 39–51.

Greenlee, R.T., Murray, T., Bolden, S., Wingo, P.A. (2000). Cancer statistics 2000. *California Cancer Journal Clinic* 50: 7–33.

Haas, J.S., Dean, M.L., Hung, Y.Y., Rennie, D.J. (2003). Differences in mortality among patients with community-acquired pneumonia in California by ethnicity and hospital characteristics. *American Journal of Medicine* 114: 660–664.

Harris, M.I., Eastman, R.C., Cowie, C.C., Flegal, K.M., Eberhardt, M.S. (1999). Racial and ethnic differences in glycemic control of adults with type 2 diabetes. *Diabetes Care* 22: 403–408.

Heaven, P.C.L. (1999). Human values, conservatism, and stereotypes of homosexuals. *Personality and Individual Differences* 27: 109–118.

Hemenway, D., Shinoda-Tagawa, T. & Miller, M. (2002). Firearm availability and female homicide rates among 25 populous high-income countries. *Journal of the American Medical Women's Association* 57: 100–104.

Herek, G.M. (1984). Beyond "homophobia": A social psychological perspective on attitudes towards lesbians and gay men. *Journal of Homosexuality* 10: 1–21.

Hickson, F., Reid, D., Weatherburn, P., Stephens, M., Nutland, W., Boakye, P. (2004). HIV, sexual risk, and ethnicity among men in England who have sex with men. *Sexually Transmitted Infections* 80(6): 443–450.

Hinrichs, D.W., Rosenberg, P.J. (2002). Attitudes towards gay, lesbian, and bisexual persons among heterosexual liberal arts college students. *Journal of Homosexuality* 43(1): 61–84.

Ho, C.K. (1990). An analysis of domestic violence in Asian-American communities: A multicultural approach to counseling. In L.S. Brown, M.P.P. Root (Eds.). *Diversity and Complexity in Feminist Therapy* (pp. 129–150). New York: Haworth Press.

Houston, T.K., Scarinci, I.C., Person, S.D., Greene, P.G. (2005). Patient smoking cessation advice by health care providers: The role of ethnicity, socioeconomic status, and health. *American Journal of Public Health* 95(6): 1056–1061.

Hsu, J.L., Glaser, S.L., West, D.W. (1997). Racial/ethnic differences in breast cancer survival among San Francisco Bay Area women. *Journal of the National Cancer Institute* 89: 1311–1312.

James, C.A., Bourgeois, F.T., Shannon, M.W. (2005). Association of race/ethnicity with emergency department wait times. *Pediatrics* 115(3): 786.

Johnson, R.L., Roter, D., Powe, N.R., Cooper, L.A. (2004). Patient race/ethnicity and quality of patient-physician communication during medical visits. *American Journal of Public Health* 94(12): 2084–2090.

Jorm, A.F., Korten, A.E., Rodgers, B., Jacomb, P.A., Christensen, H. (2002). Sexual orientation and mental health: Results from a community survey of young- and middle-aged adults. *British Journal of Psychiatry* 180: 423–427.

Joslyn, S.A., West, M.M. (2000). Racial differences in breast carcinoma survival. *Cancer* 88: 114–123.

Kantor, G.K., Jasinski, J.L. & Aldarondo, E. (1994). Sociocultural status and incidence of marital violence in Hispanic families. *Violence and Victims* 9: 207–222.

Karter, A.J., Ferrara, A., Darbinian, J., Ackerman, L.M., Selby, J.V. (2000). Self-monitoring of blood glucose: Language and financial barriers in a managed care population with diabetes. *Diabetes Care* 23: 477–483.

Kim, E.J., Kim, K.S., Lee, T.H., Kim, D.Y. (1976). The incidence of diabetes mellitus in urban and rural populations in Korea. In Ss. Baba, Y. Goto, I Fukui (Eds.), *Diabetes Mellitus in Asia. Ecological Aspects of Epidemiology, Complications and Treatment* (pp. 41–44). Amsterdam, The Netherlands: Excerpta Medica.

Kite, M.E., Whitley, B.E., Jr. (1998). Do heterosexual women and men differ in their attitudes toward homosexuality? A conceptual and methodological analysis. In G.M. Herek (Ed.), *Stigma and Sexual Orientation: Understanding Prejudice against Lesbians, Gay Men, and Bisexuals* (pp. 39–61). Thousand Oaks, California: Sage.

Kogan, M.D., Kotelchuck, M., Alexander, G.R., Johnson, W.E. (1994). Racial disparities in reported prenatal care advice from health care providers. *American Journal of Public Health* 84: 82–88.

Krieger, N., Sidney, S., Coakley, E. (1998). Racial discrimination and skin color in the CARDIA study: Implications for public health research: Coronary artery risk development in young adults. *American Journal of Public Health* 88: 1308–1313.

Kudo, Y., Falcligia, G.A., Couch, S.C. (2000). Evolution of meal patterns and food choices of Japanese-American females born in the United States. *European Journal of Clinical Nutrition* 54: 665–670.

Lau, T.K., Fung, H.Y., Rogers, M.S., Cheung, K.L. (1998). Racial variation in incidence of trisomy 21: Survey of 57,742 Chinese deliveries. *American Journal of Genetics* 75: 386–388.

Leucht, S., Pitschel-Walz, G., Abraham, D., Kissling, W. (1999). Efficacy and extrapyramidal side-effects of the new antipsychotics olanzapine, quetiapine, risperidone, and sertindole compared to conventional antipsychotics and placebo: A meta-analysis of randomized controlled trials. *Schizophrenia Research* 35: 51–68.

Li, C.I., Malone, K.E., Daling, J.R. (2003). Differences in breast cancer stage, treatment, and survival by race and ethnicity. *Archives of Internal Medicine* 163: 49–56.

Lin, B., Frazao, E. (1999). *Away-From-Home Foods Increasingly Important to Quality of American Diet*. [Agriculture Information Bulletin 749]. Washington, D.C: United States Department of Agriculture.

Lippincott, J.A., Wlazelek, B., Schumacher, L. (2000). Comparison: Attitudes toward homosexuality of international and American college students. *Psychological Reports* 87: 1053–1056.

Loue, S. (2006). *Sexual Partnering, Sexual Practices, and Health*. New York: Springer.

Lockhart, L., White, B.W. (1989). Understanding marital violence in the black community. *Journal of Interpersonal Violence* 4: 421–436.

Lynch, J.W., Kaplan, G.A., Shema, S.J. (1997). Cumulative impact of sustained economic hardship on physical, cognitive, psychological, and social functioning. *New England Journal of Medicine* 337: 1889–1895.

Makepeace, J.M. (1981). Courtship violence among college students. *Family Relations* 30: 97–102.

Manson, J.E., Rimm, E.B., Stampfer, M.J., Colditz, G.A., Willett, W.C., Krolewski, A.S., Rosner, B., Hennekens, C.H., Speizer, F.E. (1991). Physical activity and incidence of non-insulin-dependent diabetes mellitus in women. *Lancet* 338: 774–778.

Martin, S.L., English, K.T., Clark, K.A., Silenti, D. & Kupper, K.L. (1996). Violence and substance use among North Carolina pregnant women. *American Journal of Public Health* 86: 991–998.

Massachusetts Medical Society Committee on Nutrition. (1989). Fast-food fare. *New England Journal of Medicine* 321: 752–756.

Matthews, A.K., Peterman, A.H., Delaney, P., Menard, L., Brandenburg, D. (2002). A qualitative exploration of the experiences of lesbian and heterosexual patients with breast cancer. *Oncology Nursing Forum* 29(10): 1455–1462.

McFarlane, J., Parker, B., Soeken, K. & Bullock, L. (1992). Assessing for abuse during pregnancy: Severity and frequency of injuries and associated entry into prenatal care. *Journal of the American Medical Association* 267: 3176–3178.

McGill, H.C. Jr., McMahan, C.A., Malcom, G.T., Oalmann, M.C., Strong, J.P. (1997). Effects of serum lipoproteins and smoking on atherosclerosis in young men and women. The PDAY research Groups: Pathological determinants of atherosclerosis in youth. *Arteriosclerosis, Thrombosis, and Vascular Biology* 17: 95–106.

McGinnis, J.M., Foege, W.H. (1993). Actual causes of death in the United States. *Journal of the American Medical Association* 270: 2207–2212.

McKeigue, P.M., Miller, G.J., Marmot, M.G. (1989). Coronary heart disease in South Asians overseas—A review. *Journal of Clinical Epidemiology* 42: 597–609.

McWhorter, W.P., Boyd, G.M., Mattson, M.E. (1993). Predictors of quitting smoking: The NHANESI follow-up experience. *Journal of Clinical Epidemiology* 43: 1399–1405.

Middleman, A.B. (2004). Race/ethnicity and gender disparities in the utilization of a school-based hepatitis B immunization initiative. *Journal of Adolescent Health* 34: 414–419.

Mokdad, A.H., Bowman, B.A., Ford, E.S., Vinicor, F., Marks, J.S., Koplan, J.P. (2001). The continuing epidemics of obesity and diabetes in the United States. *Journal of the American Medical Association* 286: 195–200.

North American Association of Central Cancer Registries UDSC. (1996). *Final Report: Subcommittee on Methodologic Issues of Measuring Cancer among Hispanics*. Springfield, Illinois: North American Association of Central Cancer Registries.

Novotny, T.E., Warner, K.E., Kendrick, J.S., Remington, P.L. (1988). Smoking in blacks and whites: Socioeconomic and demographic differences. *American Journal of Public Health* 78: 1187–1189.

Opolka, J.L., Rascati, K.L., Brown, C.M., Gibson, P.J. (2003). Role of ethnicity in predicting antipsychotic medication adherence. *The Annals of Pharmacotherapy* 37: 625–630.

Osler, M., Prescott, E., Godtfredsen, N., Hein, H.O., Schnohr, P. (1999). Gender and determinants of smoking cessation: A longitudinal study. *Preventive Medicine* 29: 57–62.

Paxton, K.C., Myers, H.F., Hall, N.M., Javanbakht, M. (2004). Ethnicity, serostatus, and psychosocial differences in sexual risk behavior among HIV-seropositive and HIV-seronegative women. *AIDS and Behavior* 8(4): 405–415.

Peipert, J.F., Domagalski, L.R. (1994). Epidemiology of adolescent sexual assault. *Obstetrics & Gynecology* 84: 867–871.

Perilla, J.L., Bakeman, R., Norris, F.H. (1994). Culture and domestic violence: The ecology of abused Latinas. *Violence and Victims* 9: 325–339.

Pettiti, D.B., Hiatt, R.A., Chin, V., Croughan-Minihane, M. (1991). An outcome evaluation of the content and quality of prenatal care. *Birth* 18: 21–25.

Plichta, S. (1997). Violence, health, and the use of health services. In M. Falik, K. Collins (Eds.). *Women's Health: The Commonwealth Fund Survey* (pp. 237–272). Baltimore, Maryland: Johns Hopkins Press.

Ray, J.G., Vermeulen, M.J., Meier, C., Cole, D.E.C., Wyatt, P.R. (2004). Maternal ethnicity and risk of neural tube defects: A population-based study. *Canadian Medical Association Journal* 171(4): 343–345.

Rennison, C.M. (2001). *Bureau of Justice Statistics National Crime Victimization Survey: Criminal Victimization 2000: Changes 1999–2000 with Trends 1993–2000*. Washington, D.C.: United States Department of Justice, Office of Justice Programs, Bureau of Justice Statistics.

Rennison, C.M. & Welchans, S. (2002). *Special Report: Intimate Partner Violence*. Washington, D.C.: United States Department of Justice, Office of Justice Programs, Bureau of Justice Statistics.

Rogstad, K.E., Clementson, C., Ahmed-Jushuf, I.H. (1999). Contact tracing for gonorrhea in homosexual and heterosexual men. *International Journal of STD & AIDS* 10: 536–538.

Rohrer, J.E., Kruse, G., Zhang, Y. (2004). Hispanic ethnicity, rural residence, and regular source of care. *Journal of Community Health* 29(1): 1–13.

Rosenberg, N.A., Pritchard, J.K., Weber, J.L., Cann, H.M., Kidd, K.K., Zhivotovsky, L.A., Feldman, M.W. (2002). Genetic structure of human populations. *Science* 298: 2381–2385.

Ryan, D.P., Compton, C., Mayer, R.J. (2000). Carcinoma of the anal canal. *New England Journal of Medicine* 342: 792–800.

Saaddine, J.B., Engelgau, M.M., Beckles, G.L., Gregg, E.W., Thompson, T.J., Narayan, K.M. (2002). A diabetes report card for the United States: Quality of care in the 1990s. *Annals of Internal Medicine* 136: 565–574.

Schindhelm, R.K., Hospers, H.J. (2004). Sex with men before coming-out: Relation to sexual activity and sexual risk-taking behavior. *Archives of Sexual Behavior* 33(6): 585–591.

Schlosser, E. (2001). *Fast Food Nation*. New York: Houghton Mifflin.

Shaw, G.M., Carmichael, S.L., Nelson, V. (2002). Congenital malformations in offspring of Vietnamese women in California, 1985–1997. *Teratology* 65: 121–124.

Sleath, B., Rubin, R.H., Wurst, K. (2003). The influence of Hispanic ethnicity on patients' expression of complaints about and problems with adherence to antidepressant therapy. *Clinical Therapeutics* 25(6): 1739–1749.

Smith, R., Saslow, D. (2002). Breast cancer. In G.M. Wingood, R.J. DiClemente (Eds.), *Handbook of Women's Sexual and Reproductive Health* (pp. 345–365). New York: Kluwer Academic/Plenum Publishers.

Sorenson, S.B., Telles, C.A. (1991). Self-reports of spousal violence in a Mexican-American and non-Hispanic white population. *Violence and Victims* 6: 3–15.

Sorenson, S.B., Upchurch, D.M. & Shen, H. (1996). Violence and injury in marital arguments: Risk patterns and gender differences. *American Journal of Public Health* 86: 35–40.

Span, S.A., Vidal, L.A. (2003). Cross-cultural differences in female university students' attitudes towards homosexuals: A preliminary study. *Psychological Reports* 92(2): 566–572.

Stark, E. (1990). Rethinking homicide, violence, race, and politics of gender. *International Journal of Health Services* 20: 3–26.

Steinmetz, K.A., Potter, J.D. (1991). Vegetables, fruit, and cancer. I. Epidemiology. *Cancer Causes and Control* 2: 325–357.

Stewart, B., Kleihues, P. (Eds.). (2003). *World Cancer Report*. Lyon, France: IARC Press.

Straus, M.A. & Smith, C. (1990). Family patterns and child abuse. In M.A. Straus, R.J. Gelles (Eds.). *Physical Violence in American Families: Risk Factor Adaptations to Violence in 8,145 Families* (pp. 245–261). New Brunswick, New Jersey: Transaction Publishers.

Sugarman, J.R., Dennis, L.K., White, E. (1994). Cancer survival among American Indians in western Washington state (United States). *Cancer Causes and Control* 5: 440–448.

Sundquist, J., Winkleby, M. (2000). Country of birth, acculturation status and abdominal obesity in a national sample of Mexican-Americans women and men. *International Journal of Epidemiology* 29: 470–477.

Tippett, K., Cleveland, L. (1999). How current diets stack up—comparison with dietary guidelines. In E. Frazao (Ed.), *America's Eating Habits: Changes and Consequences* (pp. 59–63). [Agriculture Information Bulletin 749]. Washington, D.C: United States Department of Agriculture.

Torres, S. (1991). A comparison of wife abuse between two cultures: Perceptions, attitudes, nature, and extent. *Issues in Mental Health Nursing: Psychiatric Nursing for the 90s: New Concepts, New Therapies* 12: 113–131.

Trosclair, A., Husten, C., Pederson, L., Dhillon, I. (2002). Cigarette smoking among adults—United States, 2000. *Morbidity and Mortality Weekly Reports* 51(29): 642–645.

Tull, E.S., Chambers, E.C. (2001). Internalized racism is associated with glucose intolerance among Black Americans in the U.S. Virgin Islands (letter). *Diabetes Care* 24: 1498.

United States Department of Health and Human Services. (1990). *The Health Benefits of Smoking Cessation: A Report of the Surgeon General* [DHHS Publication No. 90-8416]. Washington, D.C.: Government Printing Office.

United States Department of Health and Human Services. (2001). *Women and Smoking: A Report of the Surgeon General.* Rockville, Maryland: United States Department of Health and Human Services, Office of the Surgeon General.

United States Department of Health and Human Services. (1998). *Tobacco Use among U.S. Racial/Ethnic Minority Groups.* Washington, D.C.: Government Printing Office.

Van Ryn, M., Burke, J. (2000). The effect of patient race and socio-economic status on physicians' perceptions of patients. *Social Science and Medicine* 50: 813–828.

Vonderheid, S.C., Montgomery, K.S., Norr, K.F. (2003). Ethnicity and prenatal health promotion content. *Western Journal of Nursing Research* 25(4): 388–404.

Wagenknecht, L.E., Manolio, T.A., Lewis, C.E., Perkins, L.L., Lando, H.A., Hulley, S.B. (1993). Race and education in relation to stopping smoking in the US: The CARDIA study. *Tobacco Control* 2: 286–292.

Ward, K.D., Klesges, R.C., Zbikowski, S.M., Bliss, R.E., Garvey, A.J. (1997). Gender differences in the outcome of an unaided smoking cessation attempt. *Addiction Behavior* 22: 1–13.

Weatherspoon, L.J., Kumanyika, S.K., Ludlow, R., Schatz, D. (1994). Glycemic control in a sample of black and white clinic patients with NIDDM. *Diabetes Care* 17: 1148–1153.

Weech-Maldonado, R., Morales, L.S., Elliott, M., Spritzer, K., Marshall, G., Hays, R.D. (2003). Race/ethnicity, language, and patients' assessments of care in Medicaid managed care. *Health Services Research* 38(3): 789–807.

Wetter, D.W., Kenford, S.L., Smith, S.S., Fiore, M.C., Jorenby, D.E., Baker, T.B. (1999). Gender differences in smoking cessation. *Journal of Consulting and Clinical Psychology* 67: 555–562.

Wold, C., Seage, G.R., III, Lenderking, W.R., Mayer, K.H., Cai, B., Heeren, T., Golstein, R. (1998). Unsafe sex in men who have sex with both men and women. *Journal of Acquired Immune Deficiency Syndromes & Human Retrovirology* 17(4): 361–367.

Wu, Z., Noh, S., Kaspar, V., Schimmele, C.M. (2003). Race, ethnicity, and depression in Canadian society. *Journal of Health and Social Behavior* 44 (Sept.): 426–441.

Young, L., Nestle, M. (2002). The contribution of expanding portion sizes to the US obesity epidemic. *American Journal of Public Health* 92: 246–249.

Xie, B., Gilliland, F.D., Li, Y.F., Rockett, H.R.H. (2003). Effects of ethnicity, family income, and education on dietary intake among adolescents. *Preventive Medicine* 36: 30–40.

Zaloznik, A.J. (1997). Breast cancer stage at diagnosis: Caucasians versus Hispanics. *Breast Cancer Research and Treatment* 42: 121–124.

Part III
Assessing Gender, Ethnicity, and Related Constructs

6
Measures of Ethnicity, Ethnic Identification, Acculturation, and Immigration Status

Measures of Ethnic and Racial Identity and Identification

Key Points

Numerous systems exist for the classification of race and ethnicity and for the assessment of ethnic and racial identification. A number of the classification systems have been discussed in chapter 3 in conjunction with the classification systems that have been used in the past by the United States government for census purposes, and that discussion will not be repeated here.

Instead, this chapter provides a description of various instruments used to assess racial and ethnic identity. This is by no means a comprehensive listing of these tools but is intended, instead, to provide the reader with examples of instruments that can be used as they are or that can serve as a guide to the development of instruments for a particular study.

In reviewing these tools, it is important to remember that some instruments have been formulated for use with specific populations and may not be appropriate for use with other groups without revision and reassessment of their reliability and validity. Unfortunately, many of these instruments have not been subject to rigorous evaluation for reliability and validity.

Yanow (2003: 211) has proposed that researchers utilize a series of questions for the evaluation of ethnicity that can be utilized across populations, regardless of their origin. These questions are as follows:

- What continent(s) did your ancestors come from? Specify the generation.
- What country(ies) did your ancestors come from? Specify the generation.
- What region(s) did your ancestors come from? Specify the generation.
- What was the birthplace of your ____ (list family kinships terms, e.g. "mother," "father," "spouse/partner," "first cousin," "mother's mother's mother")
- What is/are your cultural heritage/s?
- What languages are spoken in your home, and by whom (identify by kinship terms)? What languages do you speak?

Unfortunately, these questions have not been evaluated for their reliability and validity. Additionally, although the responses may provide insight as to an individual's ethnicity, they do not necessarily indicate how an individual may self-identify in terms of ethnicity as, for instance, when the individual's parents and earlier generations hail from different countries. In reviewing the measures indicated in Table 7, it is important to reflect on their usefulness as measures of ethnicity/race or of ethnic/racial identification.

Measures of Immigration Status

Key Points

Numerous methodological issues exist with regard to measures reported in the literature to assess immigration status. First, in general, instruments to determine immigration status have not been assessed for their reliability or validity (Loue and Bunce, 1999). This is particularly problematic because definitions of "immigrant" vary across studies, making cross-study comparisons difficult and further complicating assessments of validity. Second, few, if any, instruments conceive of immigration status as a changing value but, instead, view it as a static characteristic. This assumption may be inappropriate, depending upon the nature of the study. As an example, it may be critical to assess changes in immigration status over time if one is conducting a longitudinal study of when and how individuals utilize health care. It is unclear to what extent any of the instruments reviewed here are able to detect changes in immigration status over time. Finally, almost no data are available with regard to the field performance of instruments used to assess immigration status, including refusal rates, reliability and validity, the time required for administration, and the preferred method of administration, such as in-person interview versus written survey.

Loue and Bunce (1999) have formulated several suggestions for assessing immigration status in the context of health research, following an extensive review of the literature. First, the development of the instrument must consider the level of knowledge and sophistication of the respondent. Most individuals can indicate where they were born; this allows the investigator to distinguish, in most cases, between citizens and noncitizens. However, individuals may or may not be aware of their specific immigration designation, particularly if the law is in flux at the time of the assessment.

Second, the political and social climate at the particular time of the assessment must be considered, because this may impact both how questions relating to immigration status should be framed and how respondents will answer. It has been reported that individuals may delay seeking care if they fear being reported to immigration authorities; it is unclear to what extent individuals may refuse to divulge immigration status or may inaccurately report their immigration status in response to a more restrictive social climate or more stringent enforcement of immigration laws.

TABLE 7. Summary table of selected measures of ethnic and racial identity and identification

Instrument	Features	Properties	Sample items
Adolescent Survey of Black Life (Resnicow, Soler, Braithwaite, Selassie, and Smith, 1999)	Questionnaire consisting of 18 items focusing on 3 domains (attitudes about being black and things black, attitudes towards whites, and perceptions of racism) that utilizes a 4-point Likert scale	Alpha coefficients range from .53 to .81, depending upon domain and sample	My parents are proud to be Black. White people still owe us something because of slavery.
Bazargan Ethnic Identity Index (BEII)	Instrument consisting of 11 items in 4 parts: ethnic self-identification, ethnic preference, ethnic constancy, and ethnic diversity. Respondents are asked to select an answer from a preconstructed listing of ethnic groups.		If I could choose, I would be (check only one) a. African American b. White c. Hispanic d. Native Hawaiian e. Asian f. Native American, American Indian g. Mixed race/biracial (For example African American and Hispanic) h. Other
Ethnic Identity Scale (Umaña-Taylor, Yazedjian, and Bámaca-Gómez, 2004)	Instrument assesses 3 domains of ethnic identity formation: exploration, resolution, and affirmation.		
Ethnicity and Intellectual Life Survey (Banks, 1996)	Survey consisting of 3 sections that focus on demographic data, views of intellectualism, and attitudes towards own ethnic group and relations		In your work, you accept a special responsibility to your racial or ethnic group. 1. strongly agree 2. agree 3. in doubt 4. disagree 5. strongly disagree
Multigroup Ethnic Identity Measure (MEIM) (Phinney, 1992)	A 22-item instrument comprising two factors, ethnic identity search and affirmation, belonging, and commitment, that is designed to measure	Good internal reliability with alpha coefficients >.80 on both subscales (Corcoran, 2000).	I have spent time trying to find out about my ethnic group, such as its history, traditions, and customs.

(Continued)

TABLE 7. (Continued)

Instrument	Features	Properties	Sample items
	ethnic identity. The first factor has been characterized as developmental and cognitive and the second as affective. Scoring requires summing all items in each subscale and the total scale and dividing by the number of each items on each subscale and the total number of items. Higher scores suggest stronger ethnic identity.	In study with immigrant Chinese individuals in Canada, alpha coefficient for total scale was .90 and .93 (Kester and Marshall, 2003).	1 = strongly disagree 2 = disagree 3 = agree 4 = strongly agree
Office for National Statistics (Britain) (2002)			White • British • Irish • Other white Mixed • White and black • Caribbean • White and black African • White and Asian • Other mixed Asian or Asian British • Indian • Pakistani • Bangladeshi • Other Asian Black or black British • Black Caribbean • Black African • Other black Chinese or other ethnic group • Chinese Other ethnic group
Orthogonal Cultural Identification Scale (Oetting, Swaim, and Chiarella, 1998)	Utilized with American Indian and Mexican American adolescents, a 6-item Likert-scale (scored from 1 = not at all to 4 = a lot) that assesses how close respondents feel to a particular culture		Do you live by or follow • an American Indian way of life • a white American or Anglo way of life • a Mexican American way of life

Sampling strategies and data collection strategies have not been evaluated, in general, with respect to their efficiency or effectiveness. Consequently, it is advisable to assess these issues prior to utilizing a particular instrument in the context of a specific study.

Finally, the usefulness of a particular approach to assessing immigration status will vary depending upon the purpose of the study. For instance, if one is interested in utilization of health care, it may be important to know individuals' legal status as this in itself may erect barriers to access. However, a study focusing on knowledge of how HIV is transmitted and how transmission is prevented may find it more relevant to focus on the number of years an individual has been in the United States and/or the proportion of the individual's life that has been spent inside and outside of the U.S.

A Review of Existing Measures

Table 8 provides a summary of selected instruments that have been utilized in the published literature to assess immigration status. Each of these instruments was available directly from public sources or from the study investigators in conjunction with an earlier study of mechanisms to assess immigration status (Loue and Bunce, 1999). Most have not been evaluated for reliability or validity. In most cases, the response rate in the field is not known. In almost all cases, these assessment tools were utilized in cross-sectional studies, so that it is unknown how well they would detect changes in immigration over time if administered periodically.

Measures of Acculturation

Key Points

The process of acculturation may be important because, as indicated previously, increased levels of acculturation to the dominant culture may affect health for better or worse. Increased levels have been found to be associated with an increased risk of various risk behaviors and specified diseases, but have also been found to be associated with higher levels of preventive screening. Additionally, acculturation has been used as a marker of cultural orientation that, at a group level, explains differences in health according to ethnicity (Rissel, 1997). The level of acculturation may also affect attitudes towards the provider-patient relationship and the manner and extent of disclosure between provider and patient.

Many surrogate measures have been utilized to assess acculturation level. These include, singly or in various combinations, the level of fluency and comfort with the language of the dominant culture, the birthplace of the parent, the age at arrival into the new country, the types of food eaten, patterns of ethnic media use, adherence to home country traditions, participation in cultural or religious events, attitudes towards family structure and sex role organization, and socioeconomic

TABLE 8. Summary table of selected measures of immigration status

Investigator(s)/Study	Measure of immigration	Strengths	Limitations
Aroian (1992, 1993)	3 questions: • place of birth • citizenship status (yes, no) • status at time of initial entry into the U.S. (refugees, immigrant visa issued abroad, conditional immigrant, temporary resident, illegal alien, other)	Ease of administration	Static measure Does not distinguish between various classifications that may be relevant depending on purpose of study, such as various classifications of noncitizens Individuals may be classifiable in more than one category as they are constructed, inadvertently increasing the chance of misclassification
Asch, Leake, and Gelberg (1994)	3 questions: • country of birth • status as a U.S. citizen (yes, no, refused, unsure, no answer) • self-reported current status (permanent resident or green card, temporary resident, without papers, student or tourist visa, expired visa, asylee, other)	Ease of administration	Assumes some level of sophistication or knowledge on part of respondent Individuals may be classifiable in more than one category as they are constructed, inadvertently increasing the chance of misclassification
Cornelius, Chavez, and Jones (1984)	3 questions: • And now, are you thinking about getting papers? • Are you in the process of getting papers? • Would you like to get papers? • Did you have trouble getting into the country? • Would there be any advantage to you in getting papers? • The first time that you came to the United States, did you enter with papers or did you have to enter without them? • And the most recent time you came to the United States, did you enter with papers or did you have to enter without them?	Ease of administration	Helpful in distinguishing between those who are documented and undocumented; may not distinguish well between subcategories of documented individuals

Curiel, Baker, Mata et al. (1993)	Self-report (born in the United States, naturalized citizen, pending naturalization, pending resident status, other)	Ease of administration	Useful for distinguishing citizens from noncitizens; may not distinguish between various classes of immigrants
Dumka, Roosa, and Jackson (1997)	Place of birth	Ease of administration	Will not permit distinctions to be made other than between citizens and noncitizens at time of birth
Heer and Falasco (1982)	5 questions as basis for classification of individuals as undocumented, legal resident alien, naturalized citizen, citizen by birth • Birth in the United States (yes, no) • Citizenship status in the United States (yes, no) • Possession of an alien registration card (yes, no) • Year of entry into the United States • Periods of absence from the United States for 6 months or more	Ease of administration Permits distinction between citizens and permanent residents in most cases	May not distinguish well between those in the United States legally but temporarily and those who are undocumented
Hubbell, Chavez, Mishra, Magaña, and Valdez (1995)	Series of questions relating to place of birth, father's place of birth, mother's place of birth, date of birth, date of most recent entry into the United States, number of years of residence in the United States, current immigration status (legal permanent resident, without papers, no papers but requested permanent residence, no papers but requested work permit, no papers but requested political asylum, United States citizen, temporary protected status, political asylee/refugee, other), intent to remain in the United States permanently	May distinguish citizens from noncitizens with minimal degree of misclassification because of detailed questions relating to birthplaces	Immigration categories as constructed are overlapping
Hubbell, Waitzkin, Mishra, Dombrink, and Chavez (1991)	Self-classification as a citizen, resident, student visa, worker visa, visitor visa, or undocumented	Ease of administration Distinguishes easily between most citizens and noncitizens	Limited number of categories for a variety of statuses and some overlap between categories, heightening risk of misclassification

(Continued)

TABLE 8 (Continued)

Investigator(s)/Study	Measure of immigration	Strengths	Limitations
Lambert and Lambert (1984)	Classification based on country of birth, country of prior residence, country of parents' prior residence, length of residence in the United States, length of parents' residence in the United States	Ease of administration	Inability to distinguish between various categories of noncitizens Can assess citizenship accurately only for those born in the United States because parental residence not relevant to determination of citizenship without additional information pertaining to their place of birth
Lee, Crittenden, and Yu (1996)	Status determined based on place of birth, date of birth, parents' place of birth, date of entry into the United States, status as a citizen, and reason for leaving country of birth	Ease of administration	30% general refusal rate when used in study of Koreans aged 50 years and older in Chicago area May be able to distinguish citizens from noncitizens relatively accurately
Loue and Foerstel (1996)	Utilizes flow chart to determine status	Kappa statistic = 1.0 for determinations of status as documented or undocumented	Kappa statistic for category of documentation among individuals who are documented = 0.47 Based on previously existing law; some categories no longer relevant Requires extensive interviewer training
Loue (1998)	Revised version of Loue and Foerstel (1996)	1% general refusal rate for participation in relevant study; no refusal to respond to immigration portion	Based on previously existing law; some categories no longer relevant Requires extensive interviewer training
Loue, Faust, and Bunce (2000)	5 questions: • How long have you been living in the United States? • Now, some people who are immigrants have a green card. Do you have a green card or do you have another kind of permission? • Has the kind of permission changed since August 22, 1996? • If the permission has changed, what kind of permission do you have now? • Sometimes people have permission but then it is not good anymore. Did this happen to you?	5–10% refusal rate to participate in study of access to medical care following passage of immigration and welfare reform laws in 1996; no refusal to answer immigration questions	10% of sample provided answers that did not accurately reflect immigration status Does not distinguish between citizens and noncitizens

Author	Definition	Advantages	Disadvantages
Mehta (1998)	Self-reported status (naturalized United States citizen, resident or green card holder, temporary or tourist visa, student visa, birth in the United States), number of years in the United States, year of entry into the United States	Ease of administration; May distinguish between citizens, permanent residents, and some nonimmigrants	Cannot distinguish between nonimmigrants and undocumented persons
Perilla, Bakeman, and Norris (1994)	Place of birth, date of entry into the United States	Ease of administration; May permit distinsrtaion between those born as United States citizens and those who were not	
Robinson (1985)	Self-reported status as a citizen, permanent resident, or parolee	Ease of administration; May distinguish well between citizens and permanent residents	Cannot distinguish between various classes of immigrants and nonimmigrants or documented and undocumented
Schilit and Nimmicht (1990)	Classification based on self-report of type of immigration documentation, country of origin, year of entry into the United States, basis for eligibility under Immigration Reform and Control Act of 1986, (IRCA 1986) and the status of any application for legal residency that was filed		Specific to status for amnesty and special agricultural worker status under IRCA 1986; no longer relevant
Sherraden and Barrera (1996)	Self-reported immigration status (United States citizen, green card, work permit, undocumented or don't know)	May distinguish in most cases between United States citizens, permanent residents, undocumented persons, and all others	Does not distinguish between various categories of nonimmigrants; Overlapping categories may result in misclassification
Undocumented Workers Policy Research Project (1984)	Immigration status determined based on place of birth, possession of papers to enter at time of entry into the United States, continuing validity of those papers, date of entry, and reason for coming to the United States	May distinguish well between those who are citizens and those who are not	May not be able to distinguish between various categories of persons other than citizens and noncitizens

TABLE 9 Characteristics of selected measures of acculturation

Measure of acculturation	Key features	Properties	Sample item
Acculturation Rating Scale for Mexican-Americans (ARSMA) (Cuellar, Harris, and Jasso, 1980)	Developed for use with Mexican-Americans Focuses on language preference and ability; self-identity; social, food, and media preferences; parental identity and birthplace	Alpha coefficient = .96 (Dawson, Crano, and Burgoon, 1996)	What contact have you had with Mexico? • Raised for 1 year or more in Mexico • Lived for less than 1 year in Mexico • Occasional visits to Mexico • Occasional communications (letters, phone calls, etc.) with people in Mexico • No exposure or communications with people in Mexico
Anderson, Moeschberger, Chen, Jr., Kunn, Wewers, and Guthrie (1993)	Utilized with Cambodian, Laotian, and Vietnamese individuals in the U.S. Utilizes a Likert scale to assess items contained in 2 subscales relating to language proficiency (4-point scale) and language use (5-point scale), social (3-point scale), and food preferences (5-point scale) As an example of use, instrument permits classification of individuals with respect to language proficiency as • Low on both languages • Low on English but high on language of origin • High on both English and language of origin • High on English but low on language of origin	Alpha coefficients all .76 or greater Results correlated with current age, years in U.S., total years of education, percentage of lifetime in the U.S., and age at entry into the U.S.	

Measure	Description	Psychometric Properties	Sample Item
Bidimensional Acculturation Scale for Hispanics (Marin and Gamba, 1996)	Assesses acculturation in two domains (Hispanic and non-Hispanic) with 12 items per cultural domain in 3 language-related area Individuals are scored across each domain, so that they have two scores to define the level of acculturation	Alpha coefficient for all subscales ranges from .97 for Linguistic Proficiency to .60 for Celebrations in the Hispanic domain Combined scores for subscales: alpha = .87 for Hispanic domain, .94 for non-Hispanic domain High internal consistency across groups of varying origins: Mexican Americans and Central Americans	How often do you watch television programs in English?
Cortés, Rogler, and Malgady (1994)	Two 9-item scales assessing involvement in American and Puerto Rican cultures Items focus on ethnic pride, language use, celebration of holidays, peer relations	Alpha coefficient for scale relating to involvement in American culture = .78; for Puerto Rican culture, .73	How important is it to you to raise your children with Puerto Rican values?
Cultural Beliefs, Behaviors, and Adaptation Profile (Shiang, 1998)	Utilizes Likert scale to assess attitudes relating to own, parental, and peer views of education and employment. Other items assess language use and self-identity		In my family relationships I see myself as being like people from my own ethnic group. • Strongly agree • Agree • Somewhat agree • Somewhat disagree • Disagree • Strongly disagree
General Ethnicity Questionnaire (Abridged) (GEQ-a) (Tsai, Ying, and Lee, 1998)	Uses Likert scale to assess food and language preferences, observance of traditional holidays, and relationships in culture of origin and new culture Versions available for Chinese Americans, European Americans, Mexican Americans, and African Americans		I was raised in a way that was Chinese. 1 = Strongly disagree 2 = Disagree 3 = Neutral 4 = Agree 5 = Strongly agree

(Continued)

TABLE 9 (*Continued*)

Measure of acculturation	Key features	Properties	Sample item
Psychological Acculturation Scale (Tropp, Erkut, Garcia Coll, Alarcon, and Vazquez-Garcia, 1999)	10-item scale available in English and Spanish. Individuals indicate on a scale ranging from 1 (only with Hispanics/ Latinos) to 10 (only with Anglos/Americans) their feelings and behaviors. Higher scores indicate greater affinity with Anglos, lower scores with Hispanics/Latinos.		In what culture do you know what is expected of a person in various situations? 1 = Only with Hispanics/Latinos 5 = Equally with Hispanics/Latinos 10 = Only with Anglos (Americans)
Rissel (1997)	Developed for use in Australia. Focuses on language use, use of ethnic media in native language, food eaten, and participation in cultural and religious events in native language. Each item scored from 1–5, with higher scores indicative of increased level of acculturation to country of new culture	Cronbach's alpha = 0.88 Pearson's correlation coefficient >0.86 for each item	What language do you normally speak at home? • Only (native) LANGUAGE • Mostly (native) LANGUAGE • English and (native) LANGUAGE • Mostly English • Only English
Satia, Patterson, Kristal, Hislop, Yasui, and Taylor (2001).	Two scales to assess dietary acculturation, a 10-item Western Dietary Acculturation Scale and a 5-item Chinese Dietary Acculturation Scale	Kuder-Richardson reliability for Western Dietary Acculturation Scale =.72, for Chinese Dietary Acculturation Scale =.55	In the past month did you balance yin/yang foods?

Short Acculturation Scale for Mexican-Americans (Coronado, Thompson, McLerran, Schwartz, and Koepsell, 2005)	Items coded as 0 or 1, with higher scores indicative of maintenance of Chinese dietary pattern 4-item scale abbreviated from original 8-item scale focusing on language spoken and thought, ethnic identity of self and parents, and birthplace of self and parents	Your close friends are • All Latinos/ Hispanics • More Latinos than Americans • About half & half • More Americans than Latinos • All Americans
Short Acculturation Scale for Hispanics (Marin, Sabogal, Marin, Otero-Sabogal, Perez-Stable, 1987)	Developed for use with Spanish-speaking populations Focuses on language use, media, and ethnic social relations Items on scored on a scale of 1 to 5, with higher scores indicating a higher level of acculturation to the culture of the new country	Found to correlate highly with respondents' generation, length of residence in the U.S., age at arrival, ethnic self-identification Alpha coefficient for 12 common items = 0.92; for Language, alpha = 0.90; for Media, alpha = 0.86; for Ethnic Social Relations, alpha = 0.78

status. These indicators of acculturation are of varying degrees of helpfulness, depending upon the focus of the study being done.

It must be remembered, however, that such measures do not directly address acculturation as it relates to the focus of a study, whatever that focus may be. For instance, measures of acculturation that rely on an assessment of language ability and use may suggest the extent to which individuals could potentially access services for the prevention of partner violence. However, they fail to indicate whether individuals' attitudes towards the use of such services are more congruent with those of the dominant culture or of their original culture. Similarly, an individual seeking care for depression may be fluent in English, but may avoid Western-trained physicians and seek assistance, instead from more traditional practitioners, such as shamans or *curanderos*. A language-based or event-based acculturation tool will fail to capture critical components of the individual's beliefs regarding health care that are more congruent with those in the country of origin than they are with the new country.

Measures of acculturation differ not only in content, but also across groups. For instance, an existing measure of acculturation for a Spanish-speaking population from Central America that focuses on the use of Spanish and English and the traditional celebration of holidays would be inappropriate for use with a Southeast Asian refugee population.

Summary

The concepts of race, ethnicity, immigrant status, and acculturation are intertwined. Many of the tools that have been developed to assess one of these constructs contain items that could be utilized in instruments to assess another. For instance, one's primary language may be related to both ethnicity and acculturation; an individual's country of origin is relevant to immigration status, acculturation and, possibly ethnicity as well.

It is important to remember that how one self-identifies with respect to race or ethnicity may change over time, depending upon one's own developmental trajectory, as well as the external environment, which may encourage or discourage self-identification in a particular manner. The pre-formulated categories that are embedded in an already-existing instrument may or may not reflect categories that would be pertinent to a particular population at a specified time and place. Careful evaluation of these consideration is required prior to selecting an instrument for use in a particular study.

References

Anderson, J., Moeschberger, M., Chen, M.S., Jr., Kunn, P., Wewers, M.E., Guthrie, R. (1993). An acculturation scale for Southeast Asians. *Social Psychiatry and Psychiatric Epidemiology* 28: 134–141.

Aroian, K. (1993). Mental health risks and problems encountered by illegal immigrants. *Issues in Mental Health Nursing* 14: 379–397.

Aroian, K. (1992). Sources of social support and conflict for Polish immigrants. *Qualitative Health Research* 2: 278–287.

Asch, S., Leake, B., Gelberg, L. (1994). Does fear of immigration authorities deter tuberculosis patients from seeking care? *Western Journal of Medicine* 161: 373–376.

Banks, W. (1996). The evolution of the EILS Ethnicity and Intellectual Life Survey. In R.L. Jones (Ed.), *Handbook of Tests and Measurements for Black Populations* (pp. 605–612). Hampton, Virginia: Cobb & Henry Publishers.

Corcoran, K.J. (Ed.). (2000). *Measures for Clinical Practice: A Sourcebook*, 3rd ed. New York: Free Press.

Cornelius, W.A., Chavez, L.R., Jones, O.W. (1984). *Mexican Immigration and Access to Health Care*. La Jolla, California: Center for U.S.-Mexican Studies, University of California San Diego.

Coronado, G.D., Thompson, B., McLerran, D., Schwartz, S.M., Koepsell, T.D. (2005). A short acculturation scale for Mexican-American populations. *Ethnicity & Disease* 15: 53–62.

Cortés, D.E., Rogler, L.H., Malgady, R.G. (1994). Biculturality among Puerto Rican adults in the United States. *American Journal of Community Psychology* 22(5): 707–721.

Cuellar, I., Harris, L., Jasso, R. (1980). An acculturation scale for Mexican American normal and clinical populations. *Hispanic Journal of Behavioral Sciences* 2: 199–217.

Curiel, H., Baker, D., Mata, J. et al. (1993). *A Needs Assessment Survey of Hispanic Oklahoma City Residents in High Density Areas: A Report of Findings*. Oklahoma City: Latino Community Development Agency.

Dawson, J., Crano, W.D., Burgoon, M. (1996). Refining the meaning and measurement of acculturation: A novel methodological approach. *International Journal of Intercultural Relations* 20(1): 97–114.

Dumka, L.E., Roosa, M.W., Jackson, K.M. (1997). Risk, conflict, mothers' parenting and children's adjustment in low-income, Mexican immigrant and Mexican American families. *Journal of Marriage and the Family* 59: 309–323.

Heer, D.M., Falasco, D. (1982). The socioeconomic status of recent mothers of Mexican origin in Los Angeles County: A comparison of undocumented migrants, legal migrants, and native citizens. Presented at the Annual Meeting of the Pacific Sociological Association, San Diego, California, April 24.

Hubbell, F.A., Chavez, L.R., Mishra, S.I., Magaña, J.R., Burciaga Valdez, R. (1995). From ethnography to intervention: Developing a breast cancer control program for Latinas. *Journal of the National Cancer Institute Monographs* 18: 109–115.

Hubbell, F.A., Waitzkin, H., Mishra, S.I., Dombrink, J., Chavez, L.R. (1991). Access to medical care for documented and undocumented Latinos in a Southern California county. *Western Journal of Medicine* 154(4): 414–417.

Kester, K., Marshall, S.K. (2003). Intergenerational similitude of ethnic identification and ethnic identity: A brief report on immigrant Chinese mother-adolescent dyads in Canada. *Identity: An International Journal of Theory and Research* 3(4): 367–373.

Lambert, R.G., Lambert, M.J. (1984). The effects of role preparation for psychotherapy on immigrant clients seeking mental health services in Hawaii. *Journal of Community Psychology* 12: 263–275.

Lee, M., Crittenden, K.S., Yu, E. (1996). Social support and depression among elderly Korean immigrants in the United States. *International Journal of Aging and Human Development* 42: 313–327.

Loue, S. (1998). Defining the immigrant. In S. Loue (Ed.), *Handbook of Immigrant Health* (pp. 19–36). New York: Plenum Press.

Loue, S., Bunce, A. (1999). *The Assessment of Immigration Status in Health Research.* [National Center for Health Statistics, Vital Health Statistics 2(127)]. Hyattsville, Maryland: United States Department of Health and Human Services, Centers for Disease Control and Prevention, National Center for Health Statistics.

Loue, S., Faust, M., Bunce, A. (2000). The effect of immigration and welfare reform legislation on immigrants' access to health care, Cuyahoga and Lorain Counties. *Journal of Immigrant Health* 2: 23–30.

Loue, S., Foerstel, J. (1996). Assessing immigration status and eligibility for publicly funded medical care: A questionnaire for public health professionals. *American Journal of Public Health* 86: 1623–1625. .

Marin, G., Gamba, R.J. (1996). A new measurement of acculturation for Hispanics: The Bidimensional Acculturation Scale for Hispanics (BAS). *Hispanic Journal of Behavioral Sciences* 18(3): 297–316.

Marin, G., Sabogal, F., Marin, B.V., Otero-Sabogal, R., Perez-Stable, E.J. (1987). Development of a short acculturation scale for Hispanics. *Hispanic Journal of Behavioral Sciences* 9(2): 183–205.

Mehta, S. (1998). Relationship between acculturation and mental health for Asian Indian immigrants in the United States. *Geriatric, Social, and General Psychology Monographs* 124: 61–78.

Oetting, E.R., Swaim, R.C., Chiarella, M.C. (1998). Factor structure and invariance of the orthogonal cultural identification scale among American Indian and Mexican American youth. *Hispanic Journal of Behavioral Sciences* 20(2): 131–154.

Office for National Statistics. (2002). *Social Focus in Brief: Ethnicity.* London: Office for National Statistics.

Perilla, J.L., Bakeman, R., Norris, F.H. (1994). Culture and domestic violence: The ecology of abused Latinas. *Violence and Victims* 4: 325–329.

Phinney, J.S. (1992). The Multigroup Ethnic Identity Measure: A new scale for use with diverse groups. *Journal of Adolescent Research* 7: 156–176.

Resnicow, K., Soler, R.E., Braithwaite, R.L., Selassie, M.B., Smith, M. (1999). Development of a racial and ethnic identity scale for African American adolescents: The Survey of Black Life. *Journal of Black Psychology* 25(2): 171–188.

Rissel, C. (1997). The development and application of a scale of acculturation. *Australian and New Zealand Journal of Public Health* 21(6): 606–613.

Robinson, B.E. (1985). Evaluating mental health services for Southeast Asian refugees: Cross-cultural methodological issues. Presented at the Pacific Asian Research Method Workshop and the Annual Convention of the American Psychological Association, Ann Arbor, Michigan.

Satia, J.A., Patterson, R.E., Kristal, A.R., Hislop, T.G., Yasui, Y., Taylor, V.M. (2001). Development of scales to measure dietary acculturation among Chinese-Americans and Chinese-Canadians. *Journal of the American Dietetic Association* 101(5): 548–553.

Schilit, J., Nimnicht, G. (1990). *The Florida Survey of Newly Legalized Persons.* Tallahassee: Florida State Department of Health and Rehabilitative Services.

Sherraden, M.S., Barrera, R.E. (1996). Family support and birth outcomes among second-generation Mexican immigrants. *Social Service Review* 71(4): 607–633.

Shiang, J. (1998). Measurement of culture change: Psychometric properties of the Cultural Beliefs, Behaviors, and Adaptation Profile (CBBAP). Paper presented at the 14th Meeting of the International Association for Cross-Cultural Psychology, August. Bellingham, Washington.

Tropp, L.R., Erkut, S., Garcia Coll, C., Alarcón, O., Vázquez-García, H.A. (1999). Psychological acculturation: Development of a new measure for Puerto Ricans on the U.S. mainland. *Educational and Psychological Measurement* 59(2): 351–367.

Tsia, J.L., Ying, Y.W., Lee, P.A. (1998). The meaning of 'being Chinese' and 'being American: Differences among Chinese American young adults. Summary available at http://www.ocf.berkeley.edu/~psych/geq.html. Last accessed March 20, 2003.

Umaña-Taylor, A.J., Yazedjian, A., Bámaca-Gómez, M. (2004). Developing the Ethnic Identity Scale Using Eriksonian and Social Identity Perspectives. *Identity: An International Journal of Theory and Research* 4(1): 9–38.

Undocumented Workers Policy Research Project. (1984). *The Use of Public Services by Undocumented Aliens in Texas*. Austin, Texas: Lyndon B. Johnson School of Public Affairs.

7
Measures of Sex, Gender, Gender Role, and Sexual Orientation

Unfortunately, the literature fails to reflect consistency with its use of the terms "sex," "gender," "gender role," "sexual orientation," "sexual preference," and associated concepts. As a result, scales titled as "gender" refer in actuality to biological sex; assessment instruments targeting "gender" may be used to assess sexual orientation, and so forth. Still other scales may have multiple uses.

Measures of Sex

It is important to recognize that, depending upon the community in which one is working, individuals may claim multiple sexes, genders, and orientations simultaneously. Depending on the purpose of the assessment, the measure may need to consider some or all of these dimensions simultaneously. For instance, consider the situation of a female-to-male transsexual living as a gay man. The individual can simultaneously be identified as a female-to-male transsexual [biological sex], female heterosexual [previous biological sex + previous sexual orientation], and gay man [current biological sex and sexual orientation]. The scenario is rendered even more complex if the hypothetical female-to-male transsexual is in limine, that is, has some biological features of a female while in transition to becoming a transsexual male. The portrait in this case might look like: female-liminal male-transsexual [biologically male and female], female heterosexual and gay man [current biological sex and sexual orientation]. However, an individual might also have a very different self-identity than that depicted here.

Measures of Gender

The Eyler-Wright *Gender Continuum* (1997) is a 9-item scale that assesses the extent to which males and females consider themselves to be male, female, other-gendered, bi-gendered, or gender-blended. Examples of the items include

Female: I have always considered myself to be a woman (or a girl).

Genderblended: I consider myself gender-blended because I consider myself female predominately (in some significant way) to be both a woman and a man, but somehow more of a woman.

Othergendered: I am neither a woman nor a man, but a member of some other gender.

The authors of the assessment stress that the schema "is designed for representation of the self, rather than being primarily relational."

Measures of Gender Role

Key Points

There are numerous measures of gender role that are available. The selection of a specific instrument to be used in the context of an investigation is dependent upon the purpose and focus of the study and the particular population with which the instrument is to be used. For instance, scales and measures are available to assess gender role in the contexts of identity, of stereotypes, of marital and parental roles, employment, lifestyle, societal roles, and sexual behavior. The focus of this chapter is on available instruments that assess gender role in the context of identity; other resources should be consulted for a review of measures of gender role in other contexts (Beere, 1990).

Although we now distinguish between sex and gender, many of the scales that currently exist make use of these terms interchangeably. Accordingly, some of the measures refer in their titles to sex roles when they are actually seeking to assess gender roles.

Unfortunately, we lack adequate information relating to the development and the psychometric properties of many existing instruments designed to measure gender role. This includes the method(s) by which the assessment tool were developed, the reliability and validity of the measure, and the populations in which it has been used and validated. This information is, however, critical in order to have confidence in the results that one obtains. For this reason, the measures that are reviewed below are ones for which this information is available.

A Review of Existing Measures

Table 10 provides a listing of a number of assessment tools that are used to examine gender role. The measures that are contained in the Table have been selected on the basis of several factors including frequency of use as indicated in the published literature, diversity of mechanism (written instrument, toys, photographs, etc.), and cross-cultural use. Additional details are provided with respect to several of the more commonly used measures.

The *Bem Sex Role Inventory* (BSRI) (Bem, 1974) is one of the most often used and most frequently cited measures for assessing gender role. It has been used with

TABLE 10. Summary table of selected tools to assess gender role

Measure	Key features	Properties	Sample item
Adolescent Masculinity Ideology in Relationships Scale (Chu, Porche, and Tolman, 2005)	Measures extent to which adolescent boys internalize "hegemonic masculinity" using a 12-item scale, with possible scores ranging from 1 (disagree a lot) to 4 (agree a lot) for each item	Cronbach's alpha = .67–.71 depending on grade	It's important for a guy to act like nothing is wrong even when something is bothering him.
Australian Sex Role Scale (ASRS) (Antill, Cunningham, Russell, and Thompson, 1981)	50-item instrument consisting of 10 positive and 10 negative "feminine" items, 10 positive and 10 "masculine" items, and 5 positive and 5 negative social desirability items to be rated by respondents using a 7-point scale indicating how applicable the item is to him or to her. Two different versions are available.	Alpha coefficient = .39–.81 depending on subscale and version used	Negative feminine: dependent Positive feminine: loves children
Bem Sex Role Inventory (Bem, 1974)	60 items of which 1/3 refer to "masculine" traits, 1/3 to "feminine" traits, and 1/3 to "neutral" traits, scored using a 7-point scale from 1 (never true or almost never true) to 7 (always or almost always true) to classify individuals as feminine, masculine, androgynous, or undifferentiated. A short version consisting of 30 items is also available.		
Chinese Sex-Role Inventory (CSRI) (Keyes, 1983)	51 items in Cantonese focusing on male, female, and neutral character traits, activities, and school subjects to be rated by respondents using 1 7-point scale to indicate how applicable the items is to them	Alpha coefficient = .63–.85 (Keyes, 1984)	Male character trait: ambitious Female character trait: kind Neutral character trait: sympathetic

(Continued)

TABLE 10. (Continued)

Measure	Key features	Properties	Sample item
Effeminacy Rating Scale (Schatzberg, Westfall, Blumetti, and Birk, 1975)	Measures presence or absence of effeminate behavior in males based on observer evaluation of at least 15 minutes of duration in 10 areas of functioning, such as gait and posture	Interrater reliability=.85–.92 (Lutz, Roback, and Hart, 1984)	
Games Inventory (Bates and Bentler, 1973)	3-part checklist consisting of 64 items, to be completed by the parent. Portion 1 consists of 30 games and activities for girls and preschoolers, portion 2 of 22 "masculine" nonathletic games, and portion 3 of 12 competitive athletic games		
Gender Behavior Inventory for Boys (Bates, Bentler, and Thompson, 1973)	55 items assessing feminine behavior, extraversion, behavior disturbance, and mother's boy to be administered by parents about their child		
Gender Role Journey Measure (O'Neil, Egan, Owen, and Murry, 1993)	46 items using Likert scale designed to assess gender role changes and transitions in men and women		
Heilbrun Measure of Sex Role Blending (Heilbrun Jr., 1979)	Self-administered instrument consisting of 8 interpersonal situations and 20 adjectives (10 "masculine" and 10 "feminine") describing each, which respondents rank order to characterize their own behavior in that situation. Masculine and Feminine scores are summed separately to indicate extent of blending	Split-half reliability coefficient = .66–.93 (Schwartz, 1983)	With an acquaintance you don't care much about Masculine: aggressive, assertive, deliberate Feminine: dependent, excitable, helpful
Male Role Attitudes Scale (Pleck, Sonenstein, and Ku, 1994)	8 belief statements relating to 3 dimensions (status, toughness, and antifemininity views) used to assess males' attitudes towards male roles; items are scored from 1(disagree a lot) to 4 (agree a lot)	Cronbach's alpha = .56	A man always deserves the respect of his wife and children.

(Continued)

TABLE 10. (Continued)

Measure	Key features	Properties	Sample item
Role Acceptance Scale (Berry and McGuire, 1972)	Self-administered instrument consisting of 31 statements relating to feelings about one's role as a woman, to be answered using true/false		Sexual intercourse is desirable for physical and mental health.
Sex Role Antecedents Scale (Mast and Herron, 1982)	Self-administered instrument to assess gender role of parents and self using scale consisting of 11 "masculine," 11 "feminine," and 6 neutral traits	Internal consistency reliability for men = .73 on M scale and.73 on F scale; for women, .79 on M scale and .70 on F scale	
Sex Role Identity Scale (Storms, 1979)	6 questions asking respondents to rate their personality, behavior and self with respect to masculinity and femininity using a 31-point scale for each item	High intercorrelations	How masculine is your personality?
Sex Role Motor Behavior Checklist (Barlow, 1973)	Checklist to be used by trained observers to assess masculinity and femininity of various movements, such as length of stride and firmness of wrist	Interrater reliability ranges from .58 to .96; overall, internal agreement = .80 (Barlow, Hayes et al., 1979)	
Sexual Identity Scale (Stern, Barak, and Gould, 1987)	4 items scored on 5-point scale to assess respondents on how they feel, look, and do things and their interests, rated from very masculine to very feminine	Alpha coefficient = .96 total, .85 for women, .87 for men	
Toy Preference Test (DeLucia, 1963)	24 pairs of black and white photographs of toys, pre-rated with respect to their masculinity and femininity, to be presented to children as a means of assessing their gender role identification through their stated preference within each toy pair		

diverse populations, including college students and faculty, various professionals groups, individuals with eating disorders, commercial sex workers, mentally ill persons, law enforcement officers, and clergy, among others. It has been used with individuals of various ethnicities in the United States and with populations in other countries, including several in Europe, Africa, Asia, and the Middle East (Beere, 1990).

The inventory was originally developed as a self-report measure of masculinity and femininity (Blanchard-Fields, Suhrer-Roussel, and Hertzog, 1994). The tool consists of a total of 60 items, one-third of which are deemed to refer to masculine traits, one-third to feminine traits, and the remaining third to neutral traits. Individuals are asked to utilize a 7-point rating scale to indicate the truthfulness or accuracy of the particular statement; 1 signifies "never or almost never true," while 7 signifies that the descriptive is "always or almost always true." The resulting scores for masculinity and femininity are used to classify individuals as masculine, feminine, androgynous, or undifferentiated. A shorter version of the instrument, consisting of 10 masculine, 10 feminine, and 10 neutral items, is also available.

The instrument has been subject to some criticism because of the relatively high reading level required for its use. The instructions require a ninth-grade reading level, while the items themselves require college-level reading ability (Jensen, Witcher, and Upton, 1987). Although some researchers have found that the instrument has good construct validity (Chung, 1995), others have asserted that critical elements relevant to gender role have been omitted from the instrument (Blanchard-Fields, Suhrer-Roussel, and Hertzog, 1994).

The *Effeminacy Rating Scale* (Schatzberg, Westfall, Blumetti, and Birk, 1975) was designed to evaluate the presence or absence of effeminate behavior in males. Like the Masculine Gender Identity in Females (MGI) Scale, items focus on behavior that is presumed to be associated with one biological sex or the other. The rating scale is based on observer evaluation of at least 15 minutes in duration of 10 areas of functioning: speech, gait, posture, mouth movements, upper face and eye movement, hand gestures, hand and torso gestures, body type, body narcissism, and other. The observation time is to co-occur with a semi-structured interview. All items are to be scored with yes/no responses; for instance, one items asks, "Does he flirt with his eyes?" to which the observer must indicate "yes" or "no." The total number of "yes" responses are added and used to classify the individual as not effeminate, mildly effeminate, moderately effeminate, or markedly effeminate. The scale has been used with heterosexual and homosexual men and transsexuals age 16 and older. Interrater reliability has been found to range from .85 to .94 (Lutz, Roback, and Hart, 1984).

The *Gender Role Journey Measure* was developed to assess gender role changes and transitions experienced by men and women (O'Neil, Egan, Owen, and Murry, 1993). The initial scale consisted of 46 items designed to assess an individual's experience through five phases of development: acceptance of traditional gender roles, ambivalence about traditional gender roles, anger, activism, and celebration and integration of gender roles. Respondents utilized a Likert scale to record their answers. Test-retest and internal consistency reliability have been found to be satisfactory (O'Neil, Egan, Owen, and Murry, 1993). It has been suggested that this instrument is most useful in helping individuals to identify their own sexist attitudes.

Measures of Sexual Orientation

Key Points

As noted earlier, the formulation of a definition of sexual orientation and a means of measuring or assessing it is potentially attended by significant ethical concerns due to the public policy impact that such an assessment can have. In reviewing existing measures of sexual orientation, it is important to keep the following in mind.

The words "lesbian" and "gay" may hold different meanings than does the word "homosexual," depending upon the community involved in the research. Use of the term homosexual has been decried because of its previous use as a diagnostic label and the pathologizing of same-sex behaviors (Gonsiorek, Sell, and Weinrich, 1995). The terms "gay" and "lesbian" may be objectionable to some individuals because they are believed to connote a certain political affinity and activism that many individuals may not share.

The use of the terms "homosexual" or "lesbian" or "gay" "lifestyle" may alienate some individuals and/or convey a misimpression. The term "lifestyle" implies that same-sex sexuality is a lifestyle choice, much the same way that choosing a residence might be; in fact, it may not be a choice, in much the same way that heterosexuality is not a choice. The term "lifestyle" may also be confusing because it implies a level of homogeneity among individuals with same-sex orientation which does not, in fact, necessarily exist. Indeed, it can be argued that there exists significant diversity among individuals with same-sex orientation and how they choose to live their lives. Some are partners in long-term relationships; some are single. Some have children, while others do not.

Methodological difficulties may exist regardless of what mechanism is used to conduct the assessment. Some of these difficulties are a function of the words used to describe the information being sought, as indicated above. However, additional ambiguities may arise depending upon the content and the format of the assessment.

Emphasis on a particular aspect of relationships may inadvertently result in inaccurate reporting, particularly if the investigator is unclear about what information is critical to the assessment. For instance, research has found that lesbians tend to view affectional orientation and political perspectives as key components of their self-identity, while gay men perceive sexual behavior and sexual fantasy as critical components (Golden, 1994).

It is critical that the investigator determine whether the issue of interest is sexual orientation or sexual identity, or both. Although some research suggests that sexual orientation may change over time (see chapter 4), at least some scholars have argued that sexual orientation is relatively stable and that it is sexual identity that is more likely to be fluid (Chung and Katayama, 1996). Consequently, reliance on self-reports may yield inaccurate findings depending upon when in a person's development questions are asked regarding sexual orientation and/or sexual identity. An individual who has not yet "come out" fully to him- or herself or to others may not yet be able to recognize his or her orientation and/or may be reluctant to self-identify as being of same-sex or bisexual orientation. This is particularly likely if they believe that they will suffer adverse social or economic consequences as a result of the disclosure. This may be a particular issue when attempting to assess sexual orientation among youth and adolescents.

As noted in chapter 4, the definition and perception of homosexuality and heterosexuality may differ across cultures. Carrier (1980: 12) noted that

What is considered homosexuality in one culture may be considered appropriate behavior within prescribed gender roles in another, a homosexual act only on the part of one participant or another, or a ritual act involving growth and masculinity in still another. Care must therefore be taken when judging sexual behavior cross-culturally with such culture-bound labels as "homosexual" and "homosexuality".... From whatever causes that homosexual impulses originate, whether they be biological or psychological, culture provides an additional dimension that cannot be ignored.

Similarly, conceptualizations of homosexuality and the meaning of a particular behavior may vary over time, even in the same geographic location:

In recent years, it has become common ... to speak of "homosexual behavior" as universal. As allegedly universal, this "homosexual behavior" was the same, for example, in the American colonies in the 1680s as it is in Greenwich Village in the 1980s. I don't think so. It is only the most one-dimensional, mechanical "behaviorism" that suggests that the act of male with male called "sodomy" in the early colonies was identical to that behavior of males called "homosexual" in the 1980s (Katz, 1983: 17–18).

It is also important to note that how an investigator perceives a role to be defined within a particular society may vary from the society's own definition. As an example, Gonsiorek and Weinrich (1991) compared the elements used by societies themselves and by anthropologists in describing same-sex affinity across three societies. Nine elements were examined: spiritual gifts, same-age partners, social acceptability of the behavior, gender mixing, sex with same sex partners, different-age partners, social rejection of the behavior, whether someone was always the insertee, and whether there was flexibility in being the insertor/insertee. The authors posited that, in ancient Greece, the society itself focused on four of these factors: sex with a same sex partner, different-age partners, the social acceptability of the behavior, and flexible insertor/insertee roles, anthropologists emphasized only the same-sex of the partner and the different-age partnerships. Berdaches (see chapter 4) in one Native American tribe were defined by the tribe based on their spiritual gifts, same-age partners, social acceptability of the role, gender mixing, sex with individuals of the same sex, different-age partners, and being the insertee always, investigators emphasized only four of these factors: spiritual gifts, same age partners, gender mixing, and sex with same-sex partners.

Accordingly, it is critical that the investigator consider these variations in formulating the definitions that they will be using in the context of their studies and in devising or selecting an appropriate assessment instrument. Researchers considering these complexities have recommended, as a result, that any assessment of sexual orientation be multidimensional in nature.

A Review of Existing Measures

Assessment of sexual orientation is documented at least as early as the 1500s, in conjunction with Church efforts to identify sodomites. The missionary De Pareja recommended use of the following questions:

1. Have you had intercourse with another man?
2. Or have you gone around trying out or making fun in order to do that?

Additional questions were recommended of those boys believed to have engaged in sodomy:

1. Has someone been investigating you from behind?
2. Did you consummate the act? (Katz, 1992).

Karl Ulrichs, the founder of the modern study of homosexuality, proposed the following questions to determine whether a man was an Urning [homosexual]:

1. Does he feel for males and only for males a passionate yearning of love, be it gushing and gentle, or fiery and sensual?
2. Does he feel horror at sexual contact with women? This horror may not always be found but when it is found, it is decisive.
3. Does he experience a beneficial magnetic current when making contact with a male body in its prime?
4. Does the excitement of attraction find its apex in the male sexual organs? (Ulrichs, 1994)

Mayne (1908), another investigator of homosexuality and a follower of Ulrichs, defined an urning [homosexual] as "a human being that is more or less perfectly, even distinctively, masculine in physique; often a virile type of fine intellectual, oral and aesthetic sensibilities; but who, through an inborn or later-developed preference feels sexual passion for the male human species. His sexual preference might quite exclude any desire for the female sex; or may exist concurrently with that instinct." Mayne (1908) formulated over 10 questions in an effort to determine who might be an urning, including the following:

- At what age did your sexual desire show it self distinctly?
- Did it direct itself at first most to the male or to the female sex? Or did it hesitate awhile between both?
- Is the instinct unvarying toward the male or female sex now?—Or do you take pleasure (or would you experience it) with now a man, now a woman?
- Is the similsexual desire constant, periodic, or irregularly felt? (Mayne, 1908)

A review of published literature in which the assessment of sexual orientation was discussed found that there are five basic approaches to its assessment: respondent self-identification, respondent indication of sexual preference, an inference of sexual orientation on the basis of past sexual behavior, reliance on a bipolar scale that juxtaposes heterosexuality and homosexuality against each other, and use of multidimensional scales (Chung and Katayama, 1996). Each of these methods brings advantages, but also suffers from limitations.

As previously indicated, respondent self-identification may be problematic because one's public enunciation sexual identity may change over time, depending upon one's development and the context in which the disclosure is to be made. Consequently, although the respondent is in the best position to define him- or herself, he or she may be reluctant to do so. Reliance on a designation of sexual preference is also problematic because it implies that the individual has a choice and is able to engage in romantic and/or sexual relationships regardless of the sex of their partner. In fact, attraction to members of one biological sex may not be a choice. (See chapter 4.) Bipolar scales recognize that individuals may engage in sexual behavior with males, females, or both, but assesses heterosexuality and homosexuality in opposition to each other and fails to consider diversity even within orientations. For instance, using the Kinsey scale, it is impossible to ascertain if a self-identified bisexual man is strongly attracted to both men and women, mildly attracted to both men and women, moderately attracted to both men and women, or strongly attracted to individuals of one sex and mildly or moderately attracted to individuals of the other sex.

Table 11 provides a summary of the dimensions that have been suggested more recently for inclusion in the construction of an instrument designed to assess same-sex attraction and same-sex behavior. The Kinsey scale is illustrative of measures that utilize a bipolar scale, while the Sell Scale of Sexual Orientation is a good example of a multidimensional assessment tool. Several of the instruments are discussed in greater detail following the table.

The *Boyhood Gender Conformity Scale* (Hockenberry and Billingham, 1987) was developed to assess the extent to which behaviors traditionally associated with masculinity in boys in American culture were predictive of adult sexual orientation. The resulting scale consists of five items: playing with boys, preferring boys' games, reading adventure and sports stories, imagining oneself as a sports figure, and being considered a "sissy." The researchers concluded that the absence of traits traditionally considered masculine is a better predictor of homosexual orientation than the presence of traits and behaviors considered to be feminine or cross-sexed. The instrument demonstrated excellent reliability using the test-retest procedure (.89–.92) and adequate validity as compared with scales developed by Freund and colleagues (1974, 1977) and Whitam and colleagues (1984).

The *Keppel-Hamilton Sexual Orientation Scale* (Keppel and Hamilton, 1998), which builds on the Klein Sexual Orientation Grid (Klein, Sepekoff, and Wolf, 1985, 1990), examines eight dimensions of sexual orientation and identity: sexual attractions, sexual behavior, sexual fantasies, emotional preferences, social preferences, lifestyle preference, sexual identity, and political identity. These are assessed using three different time scales: one's life up to 12 months previously, the previous 12 months, and the ideal. A seven-point scale is used to assess each dimension of sexual orientation: 1=other sex only; 2=other sex mostly; 3=other sex somewhat more; 4=both sexes equally; 5=same sex somewhat more; 6=same

TABLE 11. Summary table of suggested dimensions of assessment for sexual orientation

Investigation/Scale	Dimensions of assessment
Blanchard and Freund (1983): *Masculine Gender Identity in Females (MGI) Scale*	Behaviors stereotypically associated with specific gender
Friedman, Green, and Spitzer (1976)	Sexual behavior
	Conscious attraction
	Fantasy
	Emotional and romantic feelings
Gonsiorek, Sell, and Weinrich (1995)	Sexual behavior
	Attraction or fantasy
	Changes in erotic interests over time
	Same-sex orientation
	Opposite-sex orientation
Hockenberry and Billingham (1987): *Boyhood Gender Conformity Scale*	Behaviors in boys believed to be associated with later adult sexual orientation
	Playing with boys
	Preference for boys' games
	Reading sports and adventure stories
	Imagining oneself as a sports figure
	Being considered a "sissy"
Keppel and Hamilton (1998)	Sexual attraction
	Sexual behavior
	Sexual fantasy
	Emotional preference
	Social preference
	Lifestyle preference
	Sexual identity
	Political identity
	Assessment of dimensions at two points in time plus the ideal
	Utilizes a 7-point scale to assess orientation with respect to each element
Kinsey, Pomeroy, and Martin, 1948: Kinsey scale	0=exclusively heterosexual, no homosexual
	1=predominately heterosexual, only incidental homosexual
	2=predominately heterosexual, but more than incidental homosexual
	3=equally heterosexual and homosexual
	4=predominately homosexual but more than incidental heterosexual
	5=predominately homosexual, but only incidental heterosexual
	6=exclusively homosexual with no heterosexual
	X=no social-sexual contacts or reactions
Klein, Sepekoff, and Wolf (1985, 1990): *Klein Sexual Orientation Scale*	Sexual attraction
	Sexual behavior
	Sexual fantasy
	Emotional preference
	Social preference
	Lifestyle preference
	Sexual identity
Lesbian, Gay, and Bisexual (LGB) Youth Sexual Orientation Work Group (2003)	Individual's self-perception or self-label in relation to sexuality
	Sexual behavior
	Attraction
	Perception or labeling of the individual by others

Italicized elements indicate unique features of assessment.

sex mostly; and 7=same sex only. A seven-point scale is also used for identity and lifestyle: 1=heterosexual only; 2=heterosexual mostly; 3=bisexual mostly, somewhat heterosexual; 4=bisexual; 5=bisexual mostly, somewhat homosexual; 6=homosexual mostly; and 7=homosexual only.

Perhaps the best known of all scales used to assess sexual orientation is that developed by Kinsey and colleagues (1948). As noted in chapter 4, the Kinsey scale of sexual orientation classified individuals into seven groups:

0=exclusively heterosexual, no homosexual
1=predominately heterosexual, only incidental homosexual
2=predominately heterosexual, but more than incidental homosexual
3=equally heterosexual and homosexual
4=predominately homosexual but more than incidental heterosexual
5=predominately homosexual, but only incidental heterosexual
6=exclusively homosexual with no heterosexual
X=no social-sexual contacts or reactions (Kinsey, Pomeroy, and Martin, 1948).

Kinsey and colleagues justified their classification system and its departure from the duality utilized in the past to distinguish between heterosexuals and homosexuals by noting that

The world is not to be divided into sheep and goats. Not all things are black nor all things white. It is a fundamental of taxonomy that nature rarely deals with discrete categories. Only the human mind invents categories and tries to force facts into separated pigeon-holes. The living world is a continuum in each and every one of its aspects. The sooner we learn this concerning human sexual behavior the sooner we shall reach a sound understanding of the realities of sex (Kinsey, Pomeroy, and Martin, 1948).

It is characteristic of the human mind that it tries to dichotomize in its classification of phenomena. Things are either so, or they are not so. Sexual behavior is either normal or abnormal, socially acceptable or unacceptable, heterosexual or homosexual; and many persons do not want to believe that there are gradations in these matters from one to the other extreme (Kinsey, Pomeroy, Martin, and Gebhard, 1953).

The Kinsey scale has been criticized, however, because (1) it forces the categorization of individuals into distinct groups, rather than conceiving of sexual orientation along a continuum; (2) it measures homosexuality and heterosexuality on the same scale, so that there must be a trade-off between them, rather than assessing the degree of homosexuality and heterosexuality independently (Sell, 1997).

The assessment instrument utilized by *Kirk, Bailey, Dunne, and Martin* (2000) builds on the Kinsey scale. This assessment tool uses Kinsey scale items to assess present sexual feelings towards members of the same and opposite sex, the frequency of same-sex and opposite-sex partners during the previous year, and the proportion of fantasies about people of the same and opposite sex. In addition, the assessment tool asks individuals to indicate whether they consider themselves homosexual, heterosexual, or bisexual; to indicate whether they have ever been attracted to persons of the same and opposite sex; and to indicate the numbers of same-sex and opposite-sex partners with whom they had had sexual contact during their lives. "Sexual contact" was defined for this purpose as "any activity which made the respondent sexually excited and in which their genitals made contact with any part of the other person" (Kirk, Bailey, Dunne, and Martin, 2000). The instrument also assesses respondents' attitudes towards having sex with partners of the same and opposite sex through the use of a 5-point scale with responses ranging from "very sexually exciting" to "disgusting."

The *Klein Sexual Orientation Grid* (Klein, Sepekoff, and Wolf, 1985, 1990) utilizes the Kinsey scale to examine the past, present, and ideal with respect to sexual attraction, sexual behavior, sexual fantasies, emotional preference, social preference, self-identification, and hetero/gay lifestyle. The examination of these aspects across various points in time recognizes that one's sexual orientation is often a dynamic process.

The *Masculine Gender Identity in Females (MGI) Scale* (Blanchard and Freund (1983) is a self-administered instrument that seeks to assess masculine gender identity in females, defined as "a hypothetical factor that accounts for that covariation in male sex-typed behaviors observable within the population of anatomical females" (Blanchard and Freund, 1983: 205). The instrument utilizes multiple choice items organized into two parts. Part A, consisting of 20 items, is administered to all respondents. The majority of the items focus on the individual's childhood and adolescence. Part B, consisting of 9 items, is administered only to women who self-identify as lesbian and focuses on transsexual and homosexual activities and fantasies. A sample item from Part A asks the respondent to indicate whether, as a child, she preferred to play with boys, girls, or no one; whether it made no difference; or whether she did not remember. A sample item from Part B seeks information about the frequency with which the respondent wore men's underwear.

The instrument has been used with college women, female nursing students, and transsexual and nontranssexual lesbians. The coefficient alpha for Part A has been found to range from .75 to .92 (Alumbaugh, 1987), while for Part B it has been found to be .92 (Beere, 1990). Depending upon the resulting score, individuals are classified as nontranssexual homosexuals, transsexual homosexuals, and heterosexuals. An evaluation of the instrument's validity reported that a total of 69.4% of individuals were correctly classified using these categories.

Although the items included in the instrument refer to gender role, the ultimate classification of individuals focuses on sexual orientation. Consequently, the construct validity of the scale is subject to questions.

The *Sell Scale of Sexual Orientation* (Gonsiorek, Sell, and Weinrich, 1995) is comprised of 17 questions in four subparts that focus on biological sex, sexual interests, sexual contact, and sexual orientation identity. *Biological Sex* asks individuals to self-identify as male or female. This may present difficulties for persons who are intersex and see themselves as either of both sexes or between sexes, and individuals who are transsexual, but have chosen or have been forced to remain in limine biologically. *Sexual Interests* focuses on sexual attraction, sexual fantasies, and sexual arousal with men and with women. *Sexual Contact* asks about behaviors during the previous year with men and with women. *Sexual Orientation Identity* is concerned with how an individual identifies him- or herself on sliding scales for homosexuality, heterosexuality, and bisexuality.

Shively and DeCecco (1977) formulated a two-part five-point scale with values ranging from "not at all" to "very." One part of the scale applies to heterosexuality and the second to homosexuality, thereby permitting the independent assessment of the level of each.

Summary

In selecting an instrument for the assessment of gender role or sexual orientation, it is important to consider the purpose of the research and the research question. For instance, the instrument selected for use in a study dealing with behavioral risk may not be appropriate for use in a study that seeks to understand health care provider responses to patient disclosure of sexual behaviors.

Responses to the questions asked will necessarily be a function of the time and place that they are asked, as well as the individual's view of his or her role within the larger environmental context. Because self-identity may be fluid over time, with respect to both gender role and sexual orientation, it is critical that, depending upon the design and duration of the study, these characteristics be assessed over time or that the limitations of one's findings in this regard be stated clearly.

References

Alumbaugh, R.V. (1987). Contrast of the gender-identity scale with Bem's sex-role measures and the Mf scale of the MMPI. *Perceptual and Motor Skills* 64: 136–138.

Antill, J.K., Cunningham, J.D., Russell, G., Thompson, N.L. (1981). An Australian Sex-Role Scale. *Australian Journal of Psychology* 33(2): 169–183.

Barlow, D.H., Hayes, S.C., Nelson, R.O., Steele, D.L., Meeler, M.E., Mills, J.R. (1979). Sex role motor behavior: A behavioral checklist. *Behavioral Assessment* 1: 119–138.

Bates, J.E., Bentler, P.M. (1973). Play activities of normal and effeminate boys. *Developmental Psychology* 9: 20–27.

Bates, J.E., Bentler, P.M., Thompson, S.K. (1973). Measurement of deviant gender development in boys. *Child Development* 44: 591–598.

Berry, C., McGuire, F.L. (1972). Menstrual distress and acceptance of social role. *American Journal of Obstetrics and Gynecology* 114: 83–87.

Blanchard, R., Freund, K. (1983). Measuring masculine gender identity in females. *Journal of Consulting and Clinical Psychology* 51(2): 205–214.

Blanchard-Fields, F., Suhrer-Roussel, L., Hertzog, C. (1994). A confirmatory factor analysis of the Bem Sex Role Inventory: Old questions, new answers. *Sex Roles* 30: 423–457.

Carrier, J.M. (1980). Homosexual behavior in cross-cultural perspective. In J. Marmor (Ed.), *Homosexual Behavior: A Modern Reappraisal* (pp. 100–122). New York: Basic Books.

Chu, J.Y., Porche, M.V., Tolman, D.L. (2005). Adolescent Masculinity Ideology in Relationships Scale: Development and validation of a new measure for boys. *Men and Masculinities* 8(1): 93–115.

Chung, Y.B. (1995). The construct validity of the Bem Sex-Role Inventory for heterosexual and gay men. *Journal of Homosexuality* 30(2): 87–97.

Chung, Y.B., Katayama, M. (1996). Assessment of sexual orientation in lesbian/gay/bisexual studies. *Journal of Homosexuality* 30(4): 49–62.

DeLucia, L.A. (1963). The Toy Preference Test: A measure of sex role identification. *Child Development* 31: 107–117.

Eyler, A.E., Wright, K. (1997). Gender identification and sexual orientation among genetic females with gender-blended self-perception in childhood and adolescence. *International Journal of Transgenderism* 1(1): http://www.symposion.com/ijt/ijtc0102.htm.

Friedman, R.C., Green, R., Spitzer, R.L. (1976). Reassessment of homosexuality and transsexualism. *Annual Review of Medicine* 27: 57–72.

Freund, K., Langevin, R., Satterberg, J., Steiner, B. (1977). Extension of the gender identity scale for males. *Archives of Sexual Behavior* 6: 507–519.

Freund, K., Nagler, E., Langevin, R., Zajac, A., Steiner, B. (1974). Measuring feminine gender identity in homosexual males. *Archives of Sexual Behavior* 3: 249–260.

Golden, C. (1994). Our politics and choices: The feminist movement and sexual orientation. In B. Greene, G. Herek (Eds.), *Lesbian and Gay Psychology: Theory, Research, and Clinical Application* (vol. 1, pp. 54–70). Thousand Oaks, California: Sage.

Gonsiorek, J.C., Sel, R.L., Weinrich, J.D. (1995). Definition and measurement of sexual orientation. *Suicide and Life-Threatening Behavior* 25(1): 40–51.

Hockenberry, S.L., Billingham, R.E. (1987). Sexual orientation and boyhood gender conformity: Development of the Boyhood Gender Conformity Scale (BGCS). *Archives of Sexual Behavior* 16(6): 475–487.

Jensen, B.J., Witcher, D.B., Upton, L.R. (1987). Readability assessment of questionnaires frequently used in sex and marital therapy. *Journal of Sex and Marital Therapy* 13(2): 137–141.

Katz, J.N. (1983). *Gay/Lesbian Almanac: A New Documentary*. New York: Harper & Row.

Keppel, B., Hamilton, A. (1998). Sexual and affectional orientation and identity scales. Portland, Maine: Bisexual Resource Center. Available at http://www.biresource.org/pamphlets/scales.html. Last accessed September 1, 2005.

Keyes, S. (1984). Measuring sex-role stereotypes: Attitudes among Hong Kong Chinese adolescents and the development of the Chinese Sex-Role Inventory. *Sex Roles* 10 (1/2): 129–140.

Keyes, S. (1983). Sex differences in cognitive abilities and sex-role stereotypes in Hong Kong Chinese adolescents. *Sex Roles* 9(8): 853–870.

Kinsey, A.C., Pomeroy, W.B., Martin, C.E. (1948). *Sexual Behavior in the Human Male*. Philadelphia, Pennsylvania: W.B. Saunders.

Kinsey, A.C., Pomeroy, W.B., Martin, C.E., Gebhard, P.H. (1953). *Sexual Behavior in the Human Female*. Philadelphia, Pennsylvania: W.B. Saunders.

Kirk, K.M., Bailey, J.M., Dunne, M.P., Martin, N.G. (2000). Measurement models for sexual orientation in a community twin sample. *Behavior Genetics* 30(4): 345–356.

Klein, F., Sepekoff, B., Wolf, T.J. (1985). Sexual orientation: A multivariable dynamic process. Journal of Homosexuality 11: 35–49.

Klein, F., Sepekoff, B., Wolf, T.J. (1990). Sexual orientation: A multivariable dynamic process. In T. Geller (Ed.), *Bisexuality: A Reader and Sourcebook*. Sebatopol, California: Times Change Press.

Lesbian, Gay, and Bisexual (LGB) Youth Sexual Orientation Work Group. (2003). *Measuring Sexual Orientation of Young People in Health Research*. San Francisco, California: Gay and Lesbian Medical Association.

Lutz, D.J., Roback, .B., Hart, M. (1984). Feminine gender identity and psychological adjustment of male transsexuals and male homosexuals. *Journal of Sex Research* 20(4): 350–362.

Mast, D.L., Herron, W.G. (1986). The Sex-Role Antecedents Scales. *Perceptual and Motor Skills* 63: 27–56.

Mayne, X. (1908). The Intersexes: A History of Similsexualism as a Problem in Social Life. Paris: Privately printed. Cited in R.L. Sells. (1997). Defining and measuring sexual orientation. *Archives of Sexual Behavior* 26(6): 643–658.

O'Neil, J.M., Egan, J., Owen, S.V., Murry, V.M. (1993). The Gender Role Journey Measure: Scale development and psychometric evaluation. *Sex Roles* 28(3/4): 167–185.

Pleck, J.H., Sonenstein, F.L., Ku, L.C. (1994). Attitudes toward male roles among adolescent males: A discriminant validity analysis. *Sex Roles* 30(7/8): 481–501.

Schatzberg, A.F., Westfall, M.P., Blumetti, A.B., Birk, C.L. (1975). Effeminacy. I. A quantitative rating scale. *Archives of Sexual Behavior* 4(1): 31–41.

Schwartz, H.L. (1983). Sex differences in social competence among androgyne: The influence of sex-role blending nonverbal information processing and social cognition. (Doctoral Dissertation, Emory University, 1982). *Dissertation Abstracts International* 43: 3375B. Cited in A.B. Heilbrun, Jr., C.M. Mulqueen. (1987). The second androgyny: A proposed revision in adaptive priorities for college women. *Sex Roles* 17 (3/4): 187–207.

Sell, R.L. (1997). Defining and measuring sexual orientation. *Archives of Sexual Behavior* 26(6): 643–658.

Shively, M.G., DeCecco, J.P. (1977). Components of sexual identity. *Journal of Homosexuality* 3: 41–48.

Stern, B.B., Barak, B., Gould, S.J. (1987). Sexual Identity Scale: A new self-assessment measure. *Sex Roles* 17 (9/10): 503–519.

Storms, M.D. (1979). Sex role identity and its relationship to sex role attributes and sex role stereotypes. *Journal of Personality and Social Psychology* 10: 1779–1789.

Ulrichs, K.H. (1994). *The Riddle of Man-Manly Love.* Buffalo, New York: Prometheus Books.

Whitam, F.L., Zent, M. (1984). A cross-cultural assessment of early cross-gender behavior and familial factors in male homosexuality. *Archives of Sexual Behavior* 13: 427–439.

Index

Aboriginal Australians 89
Access to care 3, 5, 21, 43, 45, 46, 86, 91, 98, 123, 126, 132
Acculturation 43, 44, 45, 119, 123, 125, 127, 128, 129, 130, 131, 132
    assessment of 45, 46, 123, 129, 130, 132
    bicultural 44
    multidimensional 44, 46, 129
    unidirectional 44
Acculturation Rating Scale for Mexican Americans 131
Accuracy 18, 71, 141
Adaptation 44, 45, 46, 129
Adolescent Masculinity Ideology in Relationships Scale (AMIRS) 138
Adolescent Survey of Black Life (ASBL) 16, 121
African Americans 30, 31, 39, 96, 97, 98, 100, 101, 129
Aid to Families with Dependent Children (AFDC) 100, 101
AIDS: See Human immunodeficiency Virus 31, 42, 91
Alabama 32
Albania 60
Alcohol 8, 44, 88, 92, 97, 100
Altruism 64
American Broadcasting-*Washington Post* poll 76
American Psychiatric Association 4, 7, 21, 67, 68, 78
Anal canal 104
Anal cancer 104
Androgen 57, 67
Androgen insensitivity syndrome 57
Androgynous 65, 70, 138, 141
Anglo-Saxon 34

Antidepressant therapy 99
Anxiety 105
Asian Indians 96, 97
Assimilation 44, 45
    attitude receptional 45
    behavior receptional 45
    civic 45
    cultural/behavioral 45
    defined 44
    identificational 45
    marital 45
    structural 45
Atherosclerosis 94
Australian Sex Role Scale (ASRS) 138

Bad blood 33
Bem Sex Role Inventory 137, 138
Beneficence 9
Berdache 70, 143
Bicultural 129, 44, 46
Bidimensional Acculturation Scale for Hispanics 129
Birth certificates 26, 28, 29
Birthplace 119, 123, 125, 128, 131
Bisexuality 71, 72, 73, 74, 75, 149
    conflict theory 73
    flexibility theory 73
    incidence 73
    models 74
    types 73
Blumenbach, Johann Friedrich 25
Bone mass 94
Boyhood Gender Conformity Scale 145, 146
Brazil 27, 28, 37
Breast cancer 96, 97, 98, 105
Breastfeeding 90, 91
Brigham, Carl C. 41, 42

California 29, 33, 40, 93
Carbohydrates 94
Cartwright, Samuel 32
Categorization 3, 4, 5, 6, 7, 8, 9, 14, 21, 40, 73,
        96, 147
    and ethical implications 4, 5, 6, 7, 8, 9
    and methodological implications 6, 7, 8, 9
    processes 3, 4
Category errors 20, 21
Caucasian 25, 88, 89, 90, 103, 106
Census 25, 26, 38, 39, 95, 119
Center for Health Affairs Survey 77
Children 29, 32, 40, 64, 65, 67, 68, 70, 90,
        94, 100, 105, 107, 129, 138, 139, 140,
        142
Children's Health Study 94
Chimerism 57
Chinese 26, 29, 30, 31, 34, 38, 90, 99, 122, 129,
        130, 131, 138
Chinese Dietary Acculturation Scale 130, 131
Chinese Sex-Role Inventory 138
Cholesterol 94
Chromosomes 57, 60
Civil rights 7
Classes 3, 30, 34, 125, 127
Clitoris 57, 58, 67
Cluster sampling 13
Colombia 40
Colorectal cancer screening 88
Coming out 103
Communication 45, 47, 66, 87, 99, 128
Conflict 7, 32, 45, 73
Congenital adrenal hyperplasia 57
Construct validity 17, 18, 141, 148
Contact tracing 103
Contagion theory of homosexuality 107
Convenience samples 13, 78, 79
Convergent validity 18
Correlation 18, 19, 78, 130, 140
Council for International Organizations of
        Medical Sciences 8, 9
Criterion validity 17
Cronbach's alpha 19, 130, 138, 139
Cross-dressing 68, 69
Cultural Beliefs, Behaviors, and Adaptation
        Profile 129
Cultural creativity 44
Cultural disintegration 45
Cultural identification 27, 43, 46, 47
    alienation model 46
    bicultural model 46
    definition 46
    models of 46

multidimensional model 46
    orthogonal model 47
    transitional model 46
Cultural identity 43, 45, 46
Culture 15, 26, 27, 31, 33, 35, 36, 37, 39, 43,
        44, 45, 46, 47, 58, 59, 70, 74, 78, 106,
        122, 123, 129, 130, 131, 132, 143,
        145
Curandero 132

Data 9, 11, 14, 19, 26, 30, 37, 38, 69, 73, 87, 88,
        89, 90, 92, 93, 94, 95, 96, 97, 98, 99,
        100, 103, 105, 106, 120, 121, 123
    Categorical 19
    collection strategies 11, 14, 97, 123
    interval 13, 16, 17, 18, 19
    nominal 19
Depression 105, 106, 132
Deviance 5, 6, 7, 55
    Social audience approach 5
Deviance theory 5, 6, 55
Deviant behavior 5, 6, 21
Diabetes 94, 96
Diagnostic and Statistical Manual 7, 67
Diet 37, 94, 96, 130, 131
Diffusion 44
Discrimination 8, 29, 45, 87, 88, 98, 106
Disparities 3, 21, 30, 88, 93, 99
Divergent validity 18
Down syndrome 90
Drapetomania 32

Educational level 4, 41, 87, 91, 92, 94, 99, 100,
        128, 129
Effeminacy Rating Scale 139, 141
Emergency department 87, 88
Emic classifications 31
Empacho 45
England 92
Ethnic group 13, 20, 35, 36, 37, 38, 39, 46, 86,
        87, 89, 90, 96, 98, 99, 100, 101, 121,
        122, 129
Ethnic identification 35, 37, 40, 46, 119, 122
Ethnic identity 35, 36, 37, 38, 39, 40, 41, 46,
        119, 121, 122, 131
Ethnic Identity Scale 121, 122
Ethnicity 3, 4, 5, 6, 11, 12, 13, 14, 15, 16, 19, 20,
        26, 27, 30, 35, 36, 37, 38, 39, 40, 41, 42,
        44, 47, 86, 87, 89, 90, 91, 92, 93, 94, 95,
        96, 98, 99, 100, 101, 102, 103, 106, 108,
        119, 120, 121, 123, 129, 132
    Definitions 27, 35, 36, 37
    Misclassification 19, 20, 30

Ethnicity and Intellectual Life Survey 121
Etic classifications 31
Eugenics 42
Europe 3, 27, 28, 41, 42, 89, 96, 141
Europeans 28, 41, 42, 89, 92, 129
    and race 28, 41, 42
Eyler-Wright Gender Continuum 136

Factor analysis 18
Family planning 69
Far East Asians 27, 90
Fast food 94, 95
Female circumcision 59
Female genital mutilation 59
Femininity 3, 18, 59, 61, 63, 64, 65, 105, 139,
    140, 141
Fiber 94
Filipinos 29, 90
Final Solution 35
First Nations 89
Folate 94
5-alpha-reductase deficiency 58

Games Inventory 139
Gay 3, 7, 13, 15, 62, 63, 69, 70, 74, 76, 77,
    78, 79, 103, 104, 106, 136, 142, 146,
    148
    Defined 79, 142
Gender 6, 11, 12, 17, 18, 54, 55, 58, 59, 60, 62,
    63, 65, 66, 67, 68, 70, 72, 79, 94, 95, 98,
    103, 136, 137, 138, 139, 140, 141, 143,
    145, 146, 148, 149
Gender Behavior Inventory for Boys 139
Gender Continuum 136
Gender identity 59, 61, 62, 63, 65, 66, 67, 68,
    70, 141, 146, 148
Gender identity disorder 67
Gender role 17, 18, 59, 60, 63, 65, 66, 67, 68,
    103, 136, 137, 138, 139, 140, 141, 148,
    149
Gender Role Journey Measure 139, 141
General Ethnicity Questionnaire 129
    (Abridged)
General Social Survey 77
Generalizability 79
Genital reassignment surgery 67
Genitalia
    Ambiguous 57, 58
    Female 55, 57, 59, 67
    Male 55, 57, 67
Genotype
Gonads 54, 55, 56
Gonorrhea 92, 103

Greece 143
Greenwich Village 143
Guamanians 90
Guttman scale 17

Haitians 42
Hawaiians 90, 97
Health care
    access to 3, 30, 43, 45, 91, 98
    barriers to 45
    quality of 3, 11, 87
    utilization of 61, 86, 120, 123
Heilbrun Measure of Sex Role Blending 139
Hemophiliacs 42
Hepatitis B 93
Hermaphrodites
    classification systems 6, 20, 56, 57, 70
Hermaphroditism
    Causes 55, 56, 57
    Definition 55, 56, 57, 67, 69
Heterosexuality 69, 72, 73, 74, 75, 78, 104, 107,
    142, 143, 144, 145, 147, 149
Hijras 70
Hinduism 70
Hispanics; see also Latinos 26, 40, 87, 93, 94,
    95, 97, 98, 99, 101, 129, 130, 131
Hitler, Adolf 35
Hombres modernos 15, 76
Homelessness 92
Homicide 100, 101
Homophobia 13, 61, 62, 63, 106
Homosexual behavior 69, 73, 143
Homosexuality 4, 7, 8, 21, 56, 69, 70, 72, 73,
    74, 75, 78, 107, 143, 144, 145, 147,
    149
Homosexuals 4, 7, 8, 42, 70, 77, 78, 104, 106,
    107, 147, 148
Hormone replacement therapy 97
Hospitals 37, 94
Human immunodeficiency virus (HIV) 4, 9, 42,
    91, 92, 123
Hutchinson, Jonathon 56

Identity
    Core 3, 15, 31, 94
    cross-sex 66, 68
    gender 12, 59, 62, 63, 65, 66, 67, 68, 70, 137,
        141, 146, 149
    female 62, 141, 142, 148
    male 60, 61, 62
    sexual 6, 11, 12, 61, 65, 66, 72, 73, 75, 76, 78,
        79, 103, 104, 105, 106, 136, 140, 142,
        145, 148

Immigrants
    assessing status 41, 88, 90, 91, 102, 119, 120,
        123, 124, 125, 126, 127, 132
    definitions 34, 41, 42, 43
    immigration law paradigm 43
    public benefit law 43
    social science paradigm 43
Immigration 34, 41, 42, 43, 88, 90, 91, 102, 119,
        120, 123, 124, 125, 126, 127, 132
Immigration law 42, 43
Immunization
    adult
    children 93
India 27, 28, 70
Information bias 19, 20
Intelligence tests 41
*International Guidelines for Biomedical
    Research Involving Human Subjects* 9
*International Guidelines for the Ethical Review
    of Epidemiological Studies* 9
Inter-rater agreement 19
Intersex genital mutilation 58
Intersex Society of North America 58
Interviews 14, 15
Intra-rater reliability 19
Intersex genital mutilation 58
Intersex Society of North America 58
Intimate partner violence 100, 101
Iron 94

Japan 27, 28
Japanese 26, 28, 29, 90
Jews 35, 100
Joan of Arc 6
Julius Rosenwald Fund 32

Kappa coefficient 19
Keppel-Hamilton Sexual Orientation Scale 145
Kinsey Scale of Sexual Orientation 71, 147
Klein Sexual Orientation Grid 145, 148
Klinefelter's syndrome 58
Koreans 126

Labeling theory 146
Language 9, 17, 25, 35, 36, 37, 39, 40, 41, 43,
        46, 65, 86, 87, 88, 123, 128, 129, 130,
        131, 132
Latinos; see also Hispanics 92, 96, 97, 130, 131
Leprosy 34
Lesbians 3, 78, 104, 105, 106, 142, 148
LGBT 3
Likert scale 16, 121, 122, 128, 129, 139, 141
Linnaeus, Carolus 25

Lorenz, Konrad 35
Los Angeles 94
Louisiana 32, 34, 95

Male Role Attitudes Scale (MRAS) 139
Managed care 87
Marginalization 6, 8, 9, 12, 40
Marking 20
Martin, Dolly 65
Masculine Gender Identity in Females (MGI)
        Scale 141, 146, 148
Masculine mystique 61
Masculinity 3, 18, 59, 60, 61, 62, 63, 66, 105,
        138, 140, 141, 143, 145
Masochism 63
Massachusetts 93, 94, 101
Medicaid 43, 87, 100
Men who have sex with men (MSM) 15, 75, 76,
        79, 92
Menarche 97
Menopause 97
Mental disorder 4, 7
Mental health services 88, 99
Mental illness 4, 7, 8, 21, 78, 105
Mexican Americans 95, 102, 128, 129, 131
Migration 42, 43, 96
Misclassification
    Differential 20
    Nondifferential 20
Misclassification bias 20
Morocco 27
Mortality 93, 97, 98
Multigroup Ethnic Identity Measure 121

Narcissism 63, 141
National Center for Health Statistics (NCHS)
        29, 30
National Health Interview Survey 98
National Health and Nutrition Examination
        Survey III 95
National Health and Social Life Survey
        (NHSLS) 77
National Household Survey on Drug Abuse 106
National Survey of Men 74
Native Americans 30, 37, 70, 95, 98
Neural tube defect 89
New Orleans 95
Nicaragua 27, 28, 30
Nobel Peace Prize 6
Nonmaleficence 9

Obesity 94, 95, 96, 97, 98
Occluded features 20

Office of Management and Budget 27, 97, 99
Ohio 29
OMB Directive No. 15 27
One drop rule 4, 21, 26, 27, 77
Orthogonal Cultural Identification Scale 122
Osteoporosis 94

Pakistanis 97
Partner violence 100, 101, 102, 132
Parnita 45
Pauling, Louis 6
Phalloplasty 67
Physicians 8, 87, 105, 132
Pintner, Rudolph 41
Playboy 76
Pneumonia 93
Pope Benedict XV 6
Positional identity 62
Power
    and relationships
    and social context 4, 7, 29, 30, 41, 45, 61, 65, 69, 78
    statistical 12, 15, 16
Pozzi, Samuel 56
Pregnancy 88, 100, 101
Prenatal care 30, 88
Primary care 87
Prostitution 74, 106, 107
Pseudohermaphroditism
    Female 57
    Male 57, 58
Psychoanalytic theory 83
Psychological Acculturation Scale 130
Psychosexual hermaphroditism 69
Public benefit law 43
Public Health Service 32
Puerto Ricans 26, 43, 97, 102
Puerto Rico 43

Race
    Definitions 3, 5
    Misclassification 20, 30, 105, 124
    one drop rule 4, 27, 77
    pejorative system
    phenotypic system 28
    polite system
Racial identity 38, 39, 119, 121
Reactive adaptation 44, 45
Reliability
    inter-rater agreement 19
    intra-rater reliability 19
    test-retest reliability 19

Risk
    and cancer 20, 88, 94, 104
    and HIV 4, 42, 91, 92
Ritualized cutting 59
Role Acceptance Scale 140

Saint-Hilaire, Isidore Geoffrey 56
Samoans 90
Sampling
    Cluster 13
    Convenience 13, 78, 79
    simple random 13
    snowball 13
    stratified 13
    systematic 13, 19
Schizoaffective disorder 100
Schizophrenia 100
Scott-Maxwell, Florida 64
Seat belt use
Secondary sex characteristics 58, 68
Selection bias 13, 20, 78
Self-definition 3, 12, 15, 16, 40, 75
Self-identity 11, 12, 31, 69, 72, 74, 75, 98, 103, 128, 129, 136, 142, 149
Sell Scale of Sexual Orientation 72, 145, 148
Sensitivity 16–18, 31, 57
Sex
    Chromosomal 54, 57, 58
Sex Role Antecedents Scale 140
Sex Role Identity Scale 140
Sex Role Motor Behavior Checklist 140
Sexual ambiguity 55
Sexual attraction 69, 73, 75
Sexual behavior 146, 148
Sexual deviance 7, 21, 55
    classificatory model 55
    human rights model 55
    psychoanalytic model 4, 7, 55, 63
    sociological model 7, 8
Sexual dimorphism 55
Sexual fantasies 12, 71, 145, 148
Sexual identity xii, 6, 61, 65, 66, 75, 76, 79, 142, 145, 146
Sexual Identity Scale 140
Sexual inversion 56, 69
Sexual orientation
    assessment of 11, 19, 71, 78, 103, 137
    bisexuality 71–75
    causation 56, 57, 78, 143
    heterosexuality vii, 69, 72–75, 78, 104, 107, 142–145
    homosexuality vii, 4, 7, 8, 21, 56, 69, 70, 72–75, 78, 107, 143–145, 147

Sexual orientation (*cont.*)
  theories of origin 85
  and research xiv, 11, 12, 75, 78, 79, 142
Shaman 132
Short Acculturation Scale for Hispanics 50, 129,
  131
Short Acculturation Scale for
    Mexican-Americans 50, 131
  Simulsexualism ???
Simple random sampling 13
Slavery 4, 32, 34, 121
Smoking 51, 70, 88, 98, 99
Snowball sampling 13
Social norms 5, 8, 35
Socioeconomic status 21, 63, 95, 101, 112
Sodomy 143, 144
South Africa 28, 81
Specificity 17, 18, 35
Stereotypes 8, 9, 36, 40, 137
Stigmatization 8–11, 77, 78, 106
Stratified sampling 13
Substance use 105
Sudden infant deaths syndrome (SIDS) 89
Suicidal ideation 105
Suicide 105
Surveillance 65, 93
Sworn virgins 60
Syncretism 44
Systematic sampling 13
Szasz, Thomas 8

Tacit knowledge 20, 21
Test-retest reliability 19, 141, 145
Testosterone 57, 58
Thurstone Equal-Appearing Interval Scale 16,
  17
Transgenderism 69
  Definition 66, 67

Transsexuality
  Definition 66, 67
  Etiology 67
  Incidence 67
  Surgery 67
  Treatment 67
Trauma 92
Tribadism 69
Tumor 35, 57, 97, 98
Turner's syndrome 58
Tuskegee Syphilis Experiment 4
Two-spirit people 70

Ulrichs, Karl 144
United Nations 6
United States 4, 25, 26, 28–30, 32, 34, 41,
    43, 60, 61, 62, 63, 69, 77, 89, 91,
    92, 95–102, 104, 119, 123–127,
    140
Uranianism 69
Urning 144
Usual (*REGULAR*) source of care 87

Vaginal stenosis 67
Validity 16–18
  Construct 17, 18, 141, 148
  Convergent 17, 18
  Criterion 17
  Divergent 18
van Evrie, John H. 32
Veterans Administration 30
Vietnamese 97, 128
Violence 13, 40, 62, 63, 69, 100–102, 132
Vitamins 94

Western Dietary Acculturation Scale 130

Yerkes, Robert 42